Mayo Clinic
Values

❖

A Field Guide
for Your Journey

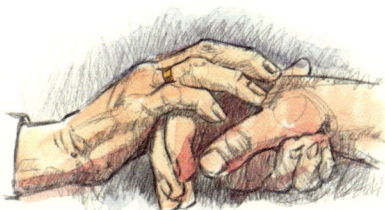

Sister Ellen Whelan, Ph.D.
Matthew D. Dacy

Illustrations
James E. Rownd

THE PUBLICATION OF THIS BOOK
IS POSSIBLE WITH GENEROUS SUPPORT FROM
GERALD AND HENRIETTA RAUENHORST

———————— ❖ ————————

*Supporting the Collaboration
of Mayo Clinic and the
Sisters of St. Francis*

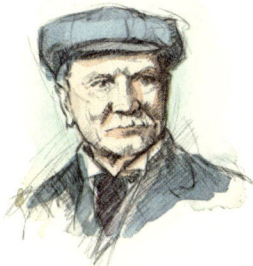

Dr. William
Worrall Mayo

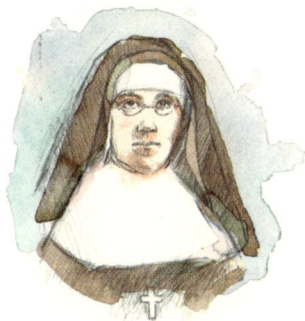

Mother
Alfred Moes

MAYO CLINIC PRESS
200 First St. SW
Rochester, MN 55905
MCPress.MayoClinic.org

To stay informed about Mayo Clinic Press, please subscribe to our free e-newsletter at MCPress.MayoClinic.org or follow us on social media.

For bulk sales to employers, member groups and health-related companies, contact Mayo Clinic, 200 First St. SW, Rochester, MN 55905, or send an email to SpecialSalesMayoBooks@mayo.edu.

Cover design by Connie S. Brooks

Illustrations provided by James E. Rownd

ISBN: 979-8-88770-295-7

Library of Congress Control Number: 2023948945

Printed in the United States of America

Proceeds from the sale of every book benefit medical research and education at Mayo Clinic.

TABLE OF CONTENTS

TABLE OF CONTENTS (CONTINUED)

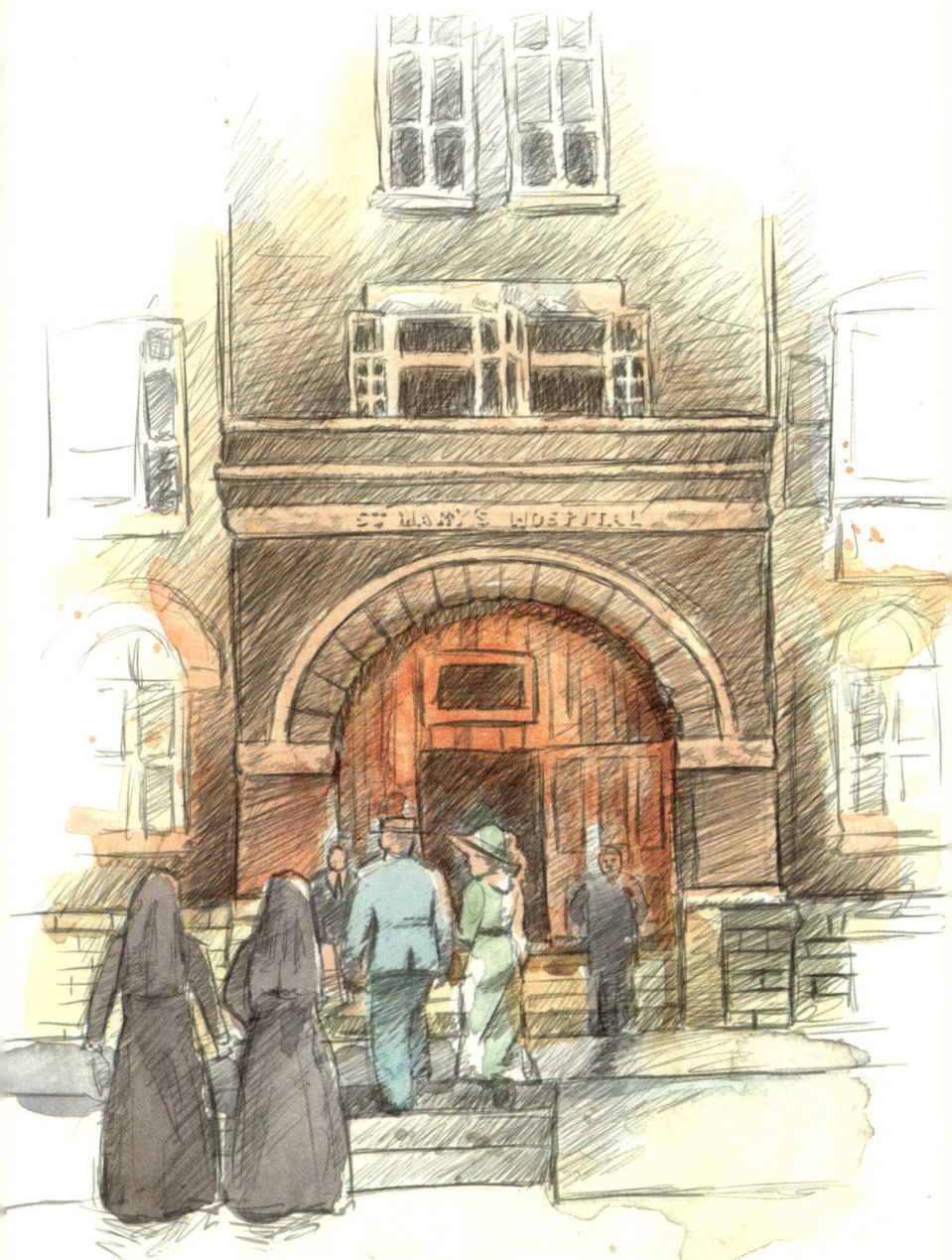

Patients came to Saint Marys
from near and far.

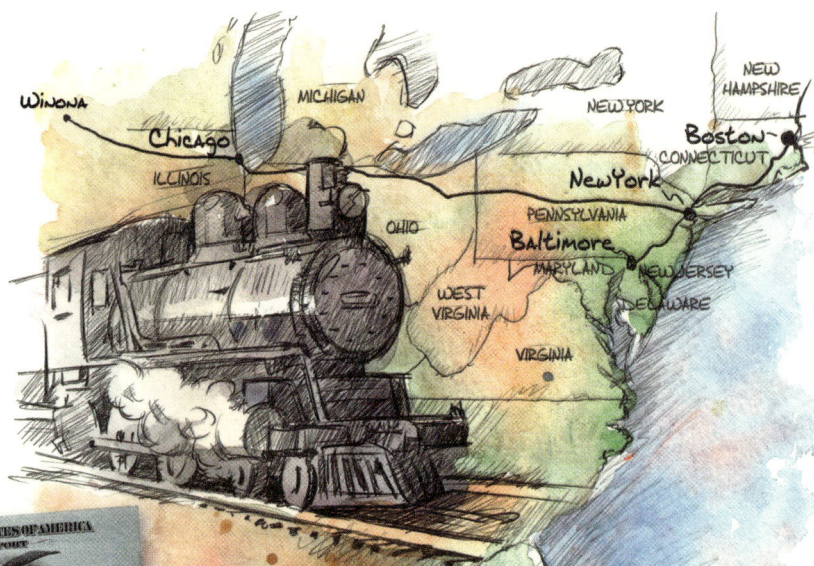

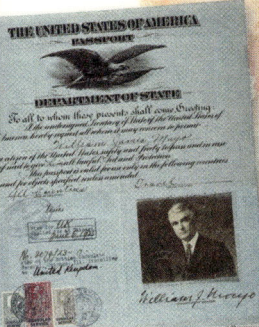

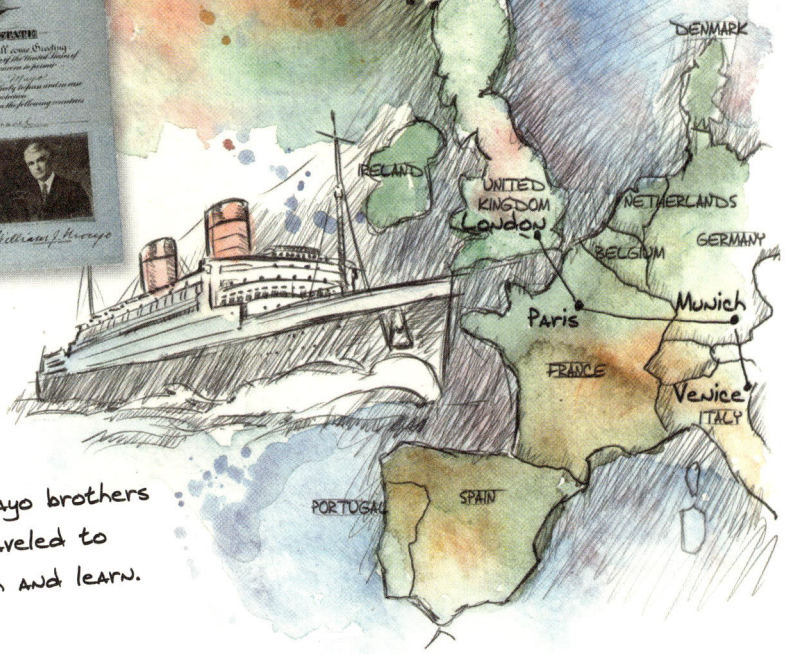

The Mayo brothers traveled to teach and learn.

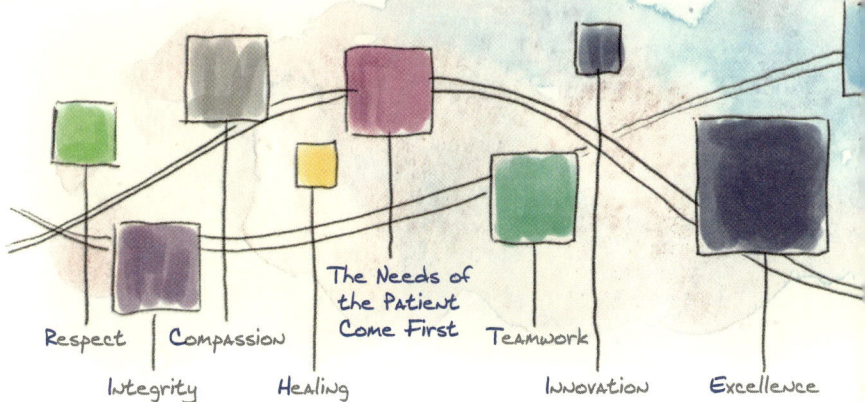

Respect Compassion The Needs of the Patient Come First Teamwork
Integrity Healing Innovation Excellence

Each generation of partners shared a common goal, the welfare of the patient. Inspired by this goal and the dedication they witnessed in each other, generations of Franciscan and Mayo colleagues overcame formidable obstacles.

The miracle of healing that happened in past generations does not end; a new generation of Mayo colleagues, inspired with the same purpose, continues to meet the challenges of today through the miracle of relationships.

— Sister Ellen Whelan, Ph.D.

The Sisters' Story Part Two: Saint Marys Hospital – Mayo Clinic, 1939 to 1980, p. 222

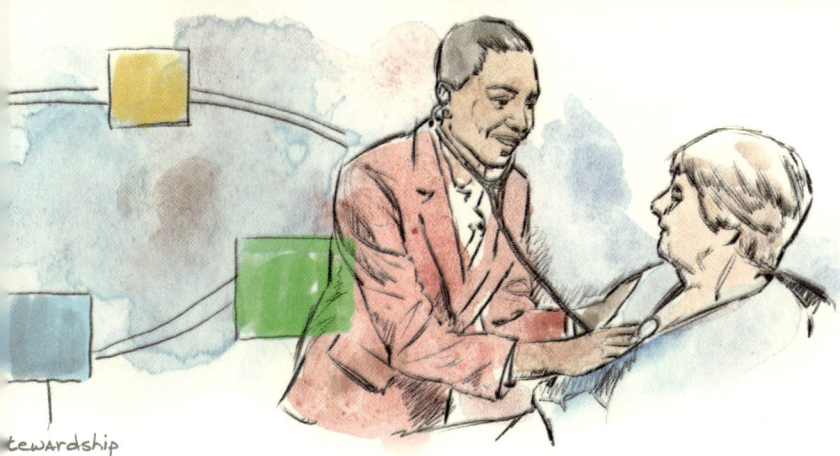

tewardship

Mayo Clinic Values:
RICH TIES

To use a figure of speech from medical science, the values of Mayo Clinic are part of the "DNA" of our organization. These values can be traced to the collaboration of Mayo Clinic staff members and the Sisters of St. Francis, along with the contributions of patients, colleagues and friends from diverse walks of life, across the generations.

This book is intended to help you discover the Mayo Clinic Values. As a "field guide," the book can be your companion at Mayo Clinic. Chapters have blank spaces at the end for you to write your own observations. A helpful way to remember Mayo Clinic Values is the acronym "RICH TIES" (page XII). At the same time, because values are organic, not formulaic, this book places them in a different order throughout the chronology of Mayo's history.

Reading this book, and experiencing Mayo Clinic as a patient or employee, is akin to going on a pilgrimage. The section "Friends Along the Journey" provides additional context about people who are mentioned in the various chapters. In many respects, they have facilitated the "handoff" of Mayo Clinic from one generation to the next. Each of us has a role in carrying forward the values and mission of Mayo Clinic.

The Needs of the Patient Come First
— Primary Value

Respect
Integrity
Compassion
Healing

Teamwork
Innovation
Excellence
Stewardship

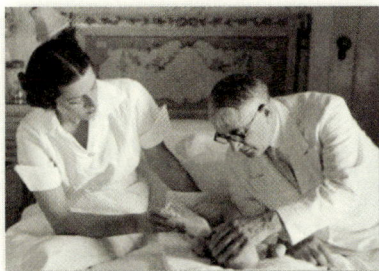

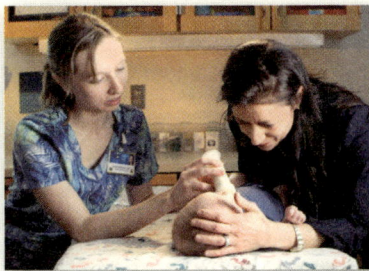

Mayo Clinic Model of Care

Along with the Mayo Clinic Values, the Mayo Clinic Model of Care defines enduring attributes of our organization.

Patient Care

- Collegial, cooperative teamwork with multispecialty integration. A team of specialists is available and appropriately used.

- An unhurried examination with time to listen to the patient.

- Physician taking personal responsibility for directing patient care in partnership with the local physician.

- Highest-quality patient care provided with compassion and trust.

- Respect for the patient, family and the patient's local physician.

- Comprehensive evaluation with timely, efficient assessment and treatment.

- Availability of the most advanced, innovative diagnostic and therapeutic technology and techniques.

Mayo Clinic Environment

- Highest-quality staff, mentored in the culture of Mayo Clinic and valued for their contributions.

- Professional allied health staff with a strong work ethic, special expertise and devotion to Mayo Clinic.

- A scholarly environment of research and education.

- Physician leadership.

- Integrated medical record with common support services for all outpatients and inpatients.

- Professional compensation that allows a focus on quality, not quantity.

- Unique professional dress, decorum and facilities.

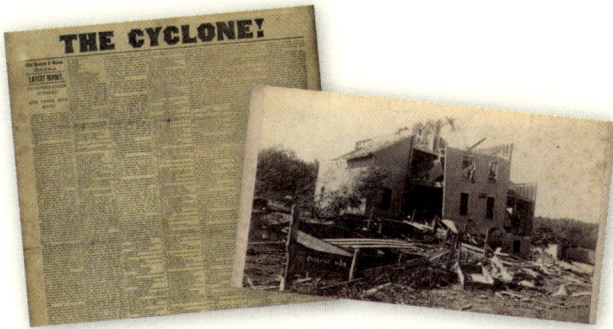

Timeline

1883

A tornado devastated Rochester, Minnesota. English-born William Worrall Mayo, M.D., and Mother Alfred Moes, an immigrant from Luxembourg, became unlikely partners in healing. Following the disaster, Mother Alfred offered that the Franciscan Sisters would fund construction of a hospital and serve as nurses if Dr. Mayo and his sons, William and Charles, provided the medical care. Hesitant at first, Dr. Mayo agreed.

1889

Saint Marys Hospital opened as an independent hospital working in close collaboration with the Mayo medical practice. As medicine became more specialized, colleagues with complementary skills joined the Mayos and the Sisters, developing a new model of integrated, multispecialty care.

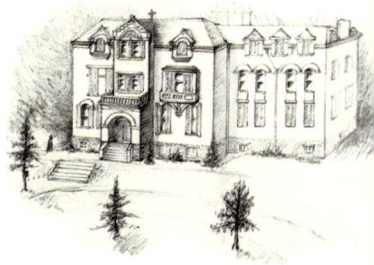

1907

John H. Kahler, a Rochester business leader, developed a unique hotel-hospital concept that complemented Saint Marys in serving Mayo's patients.

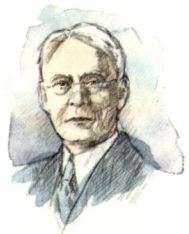

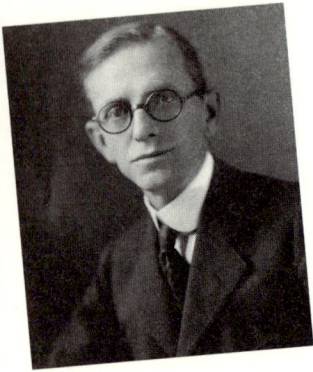

Dr. Plummer
and the building
he designed.

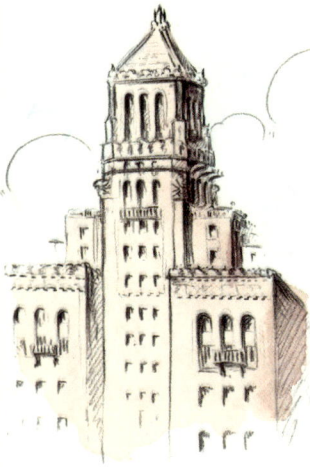

1907

Henry Plummer, M.D., developed the integrated medical record. It set a world standard of excellence in documentation and remains central to Mayo Clinic today.

1919

The Mayo brothers and their wives donated the assets of the medical practice and the majority of their life savings to establish Mayo Clinic as a not-for-profit organization dedicated to excellence in patient care, research and education.

1928

The iconic Plummer Building opened, followed shortly by the challenges of the Great Depression.

1939

Dr. Will and Dr. Charlie Mayo, along with Sister Joseph Dempsey, superintendent of Saint Marys Hospital, died within a few months of each other. With careful planning, however, they had ensured a smooth transition to other leaders.

1941-1945

As part of its long tradition of innovation and service, Mayo Clinic made pioneering contributions during World War II.

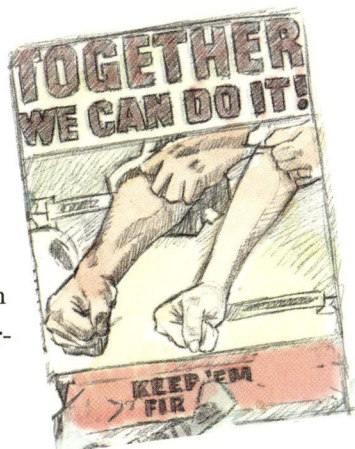

1954

As the Kahler Corporation left the hospital business, the not-for-profit Rochester Methodist Hospital filled the need for hospital care in downtown Rochester. This era also included significant contributions to medicine such as the Nobel Prize-winning discovery of cortisone and the development of open-heart surgery.

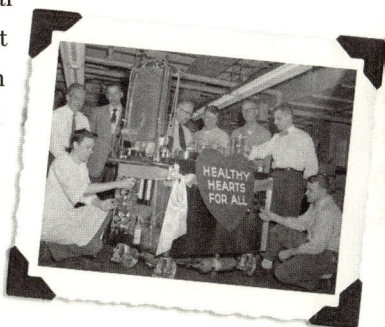

1986

Mayo Clinic, Saint Marys Hospital and Rochester Methodist Hospital formed a single governance structure, "a trusteeship for health." Mayo Clinic opened in Jacksonville, Florida.

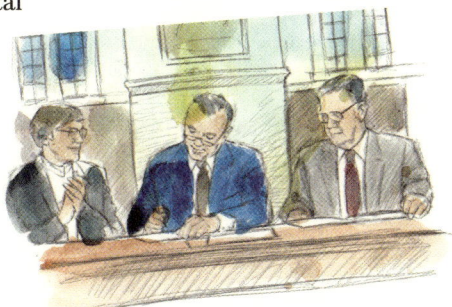

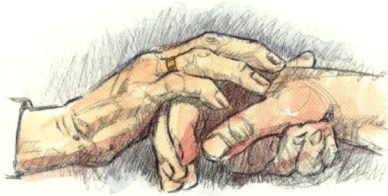

1987

Mayo Clinic opened in Scottsdale, Arizona. Mayo's campus in Phoenix opened in 1998.

1992

Mayo Clinic Health System was established to provide community-based care in the Upper Midwest.

2012

Mayo Clinic Care Network was established as a team of independent healthcare providers, throughout the United States and internationally. Members share ideals and services of high-quality, patient-centered care.

2013

Mayo Clinic Values Council was established to promote the living legacy of our values and perpetuate the Franciscan tradition on the Saint Marys campus.

TODAY

Mayo Clinic is recognized as one of the most trusted healthcare providers. Mayo's commitment to education and research advances the standard of care for our patients and people throughout the world.

References & Resources

Clapesattle, Helen. *The Doctors Mayo*. Minneapolis, Minnesota: The University of Minnesota Press, 1941.

Whelan, Ellen. *The Sisters' Story: Saint Marys Hospital – Mayo Clinic*. Rochester, Minnesota: Mayo Foundation for Medical Education and Research. Volume One: 1889-1939, was originally published in 2002. Endnotes in this book refer to the second edition, published in 2016. Volume Two: 1939-1980, was published in 2007.

Other works are identified in the endnotes to various chapters.

Annals of Saint Marys Hospital is an unpublished document about the early years of Saint Marys Hospital. Along with additional resources, it is located in the Saint Marys Hospital Archives, Mayo Clinic Hospital – Saint Marys Campus, Rochester, Minnesota.

W. Bruce Fye Center for the History of Medicine (referred to in endnotes as Mayo Clinic Archives), Rochester, Minnesota, has extensive information about the history of Mayo Clinic.

Archives of the Sisters of St. Francis, Assisi Heights, Rochester, Minnesota, documents the congregational life of the Franciscan Sisters.

For more information, please visit **history.mayoclinic.org**.

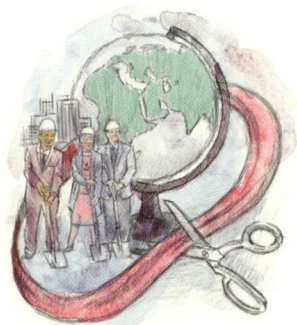

Making a world
of difference.

Mayo Clinic Values

Values

---❖---

A Field Guide
for Your Journey

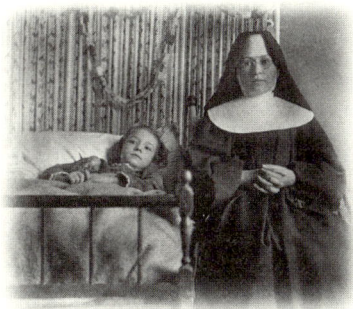

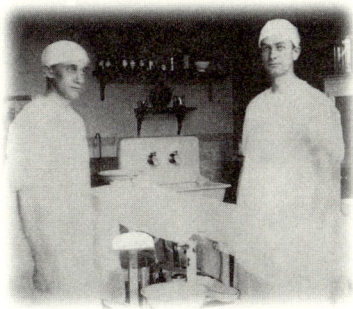

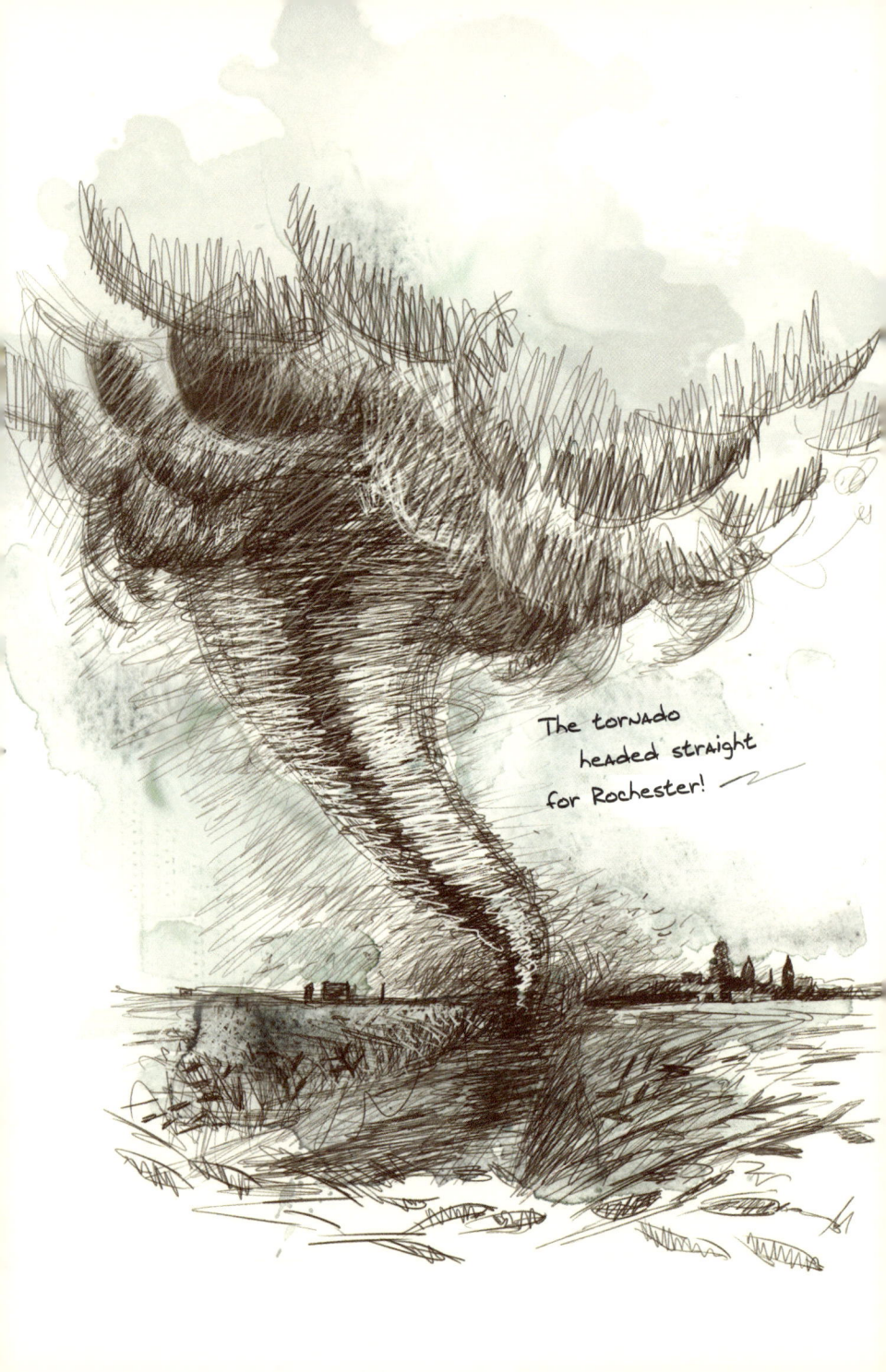

The tornado headed straight for Rochester!

CHAPTER ONE

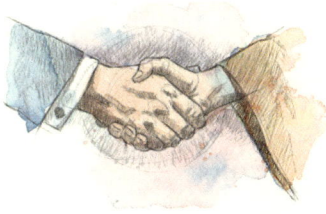

THE NEEDS OF THE PATIENT
COME FIRST

"Their duty was to alleviate human suffering ..."

— Sister Joseph Dempsey

THE MAYO-FRANCISCAN STORY BEGINS LIKE MANY GOOD STORIES. Once upon a time, a group of Catholic Sisters, working with a family of Protestant physicians, built a hospital in a cornfield. The hospital grew into a place of healing for people from all over the world. A handshake, not a legal document, sealed the partnership of the Franciscan Sisters and Mayo physicians. Working together, these unlikely partners faced daunting challenges with unwavering dedication to their primary goal of placing the needs of the patient first.

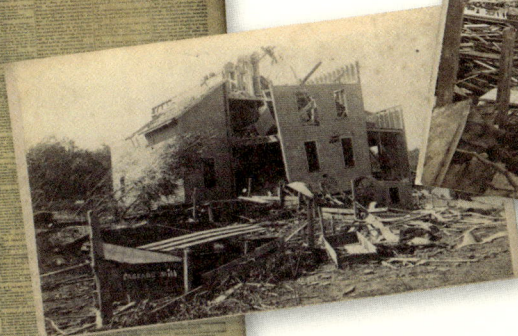

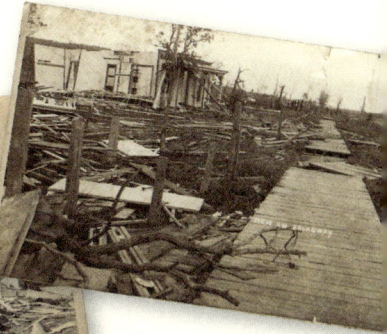

August 21, 1883

THE WESTERN UNION TELEGRAPH COMPANY.

AUGUST 21, 1883

To GOV. LUCIUS HUBBARD

ROCHESTER IS IN RUINS. TWENTY-FOUR PEOPLE KILLED. OVER FORTY SERIOUSLY INJURED. ONE-THIRD OF THE CITY LAID WASTE. WE NEED IMMEDIATE HELP.

Saint Marys Hospital, "The Miracle in a Cornfield," had its origins in tragedy. A devastating tornado struck Rochester, Minnesota, on August 21, 1883. "Rochester in ruins" was the feeble message tapped on a rigged telegraph line to Governor Lucius Hubbard. "Twenty-four people killed. Over forty seriously injured. One-third of the city laid waste. We need immediate help."

The Sisters were Appointed

to look After the injured.

William Worrall Mayo, M.D., Rochester's leading physician, took charge of medical efforts and turned the downtown dance hall into a temporary hospital. His sons, Will, a fledgling physician, and Charlie, a student, worked at his side. Dr. Mayo's first concern was the nursing staff. "Volunteers were willing enough, but they had homes and families to look after." The Mayos needed nurses who could give their entire time to the job. Dr. Mayo went to the convent of the Sisters of St. Francis. "There ought to be a Sister down there to look after those fellows," he told the mother superior. Mother Alfred Moes readily agreed and appointed two Sisters. From that time until the makeshift relief facilities closed, Sisters supervised the nursing.

Later, Mother Alfred assessed how care of the sick and injured could be improved. Intelligent and pragmatic, she typically used life experiences to solve practical problems. She was well acquainted with Sisters' hospitals in Europe and America. Her homeland, Luxembourg, indeed most of Europe, had a history of Sisters' hospitals that went back to the Middle Ages. Now a missionary on the American frontier, Mother Alfred witnessed the extraordinary contribution of Sisters' hospitals to pioneer communities. Yes, Rochester must have its own hospital. She would build one.

Mother Alfred went to Dr. W.W. Mayo with her idea and asked him to head the medical staff. "Mother Superior," he told her, "this town is too small to support a hospital." He reminded her that the public shunned hospitals as pest houses where people went to die. Further, it would be a costly undertaking with no assurance of success. Mother Alfred insisted she could build a hospital that would succeed if Dr. Mayo would take charge of it. Reluctantly, he agreed.

The Sisters earned and saved every cent they could. By constant labor and sacrifice, they raised

They saved every cent.

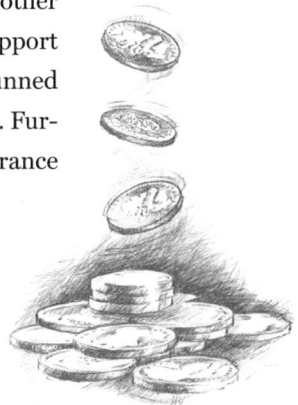

the needed funds. Dr. W.W. Mayo and Mother Alfred chose the site, nine acres, just west of the city. Saint Marys Hospital opened September 30, 1889, with 27 beds, six Sisters and two physicians, the sons of Dr. W. W. Mayo. The father, now 70 years of age, served as consulting physician. Mother Alfred appointed Sister Joseph Dempsey, a Rochester native, as superintendent. The Sisters opened the hospital "to all sick persons regardless of their color, sex, financial status or professed religion."

The Franciscans had little money to furnish wards and private rooms. They started with a few iron cots, a dozen unbleached muslin sheets and some rough gowns. Mattresses didn't fit the cots and slipped around on the springs. Just keeping the patient on the bed and the bed on the springs was a challenge. The Sisters got up at 3 or 4 in the morning and worked until 11 at night. When there was laundry to do, they got up at 2 a.m. The hospital had three floors. The kitchen was on the first floor. They carried patient meals to the upper floors as the dumb waiter was broken most of the

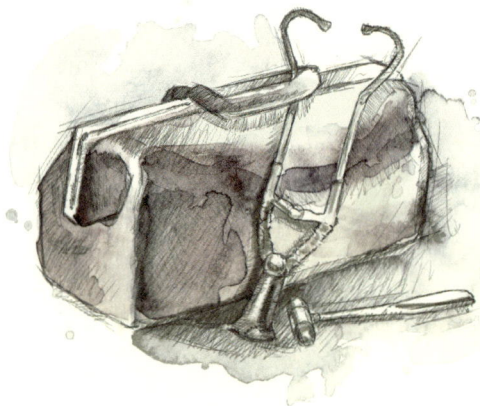

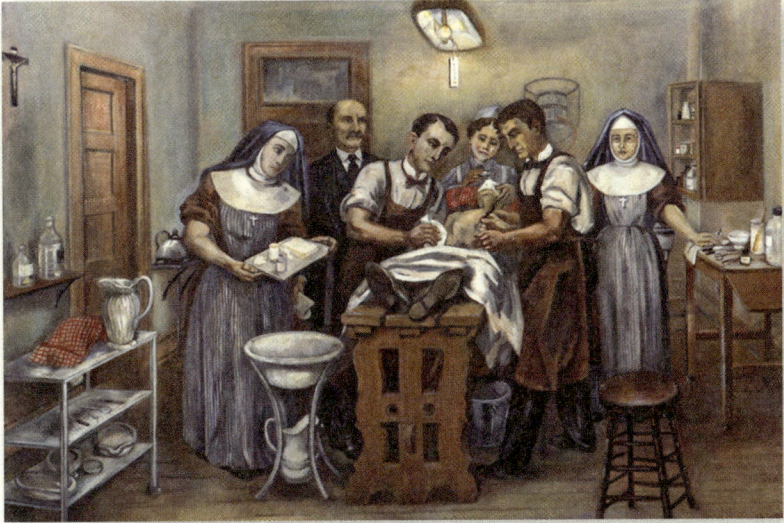

time. All the water for the building had to be pumped by hand from the basement reservoir. They carried the water used for cooking, baths and every other need from the basement to the upper floors. When the number of patients exceeded the cots available, the Sisters gave up their beds, pulled out mattresses and slept on the floor.

Demands on the Mayo brothers were equally rigorous. For the first three years, there was no male orderly. In addition to demanding surgical and medical loads, the young physicians nursed male patients who needed special attention. They each took turns on night duty.

Teamwork from the 1st day.

Sister Joseph later recalled the spirit of Saint Marys' nurses and doctors: "Their duty was to alleviate human suffering and to save human lives — and they did it."

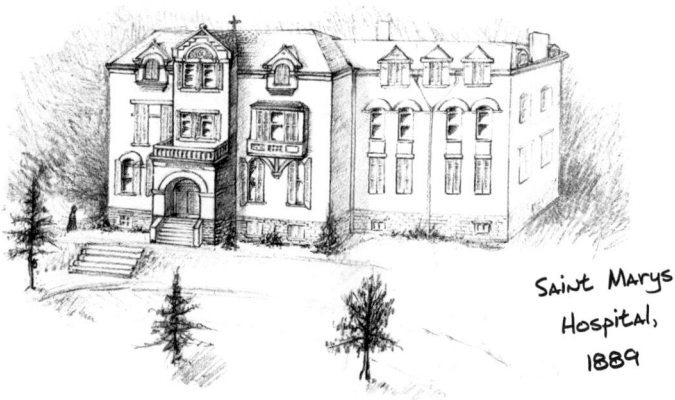

Saint Marys Hospital, 1889

ENDNOTES

Pages 3-5: **Clapesattle, H: *The Doctors Mayo*. University of Minnesota Press, 1941, pp. 242-248.** Classic account of how the tornado of 1883 brought the Mayos and the Sisters of St. Francis together as unlikely partners in healing.

Pages 6-8: **Clapesattle, pp. 252-253,** describes the opening of Saint Marys Hospital. *Annals of Saint Marys Hospital* includes the speech by Dr. William Worrall Mayo and early accounts of the hospital.

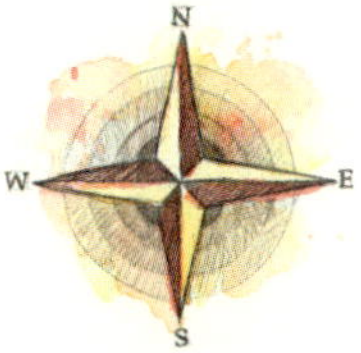

CHECK YOUR COMPASS

THE NEEDS OF THE PATIENT COME FIRST

The primary value of Mayo Clinic in our mission to contribute to health and well-being by providing the best care to every patient through integrated clinical practice, education and research.

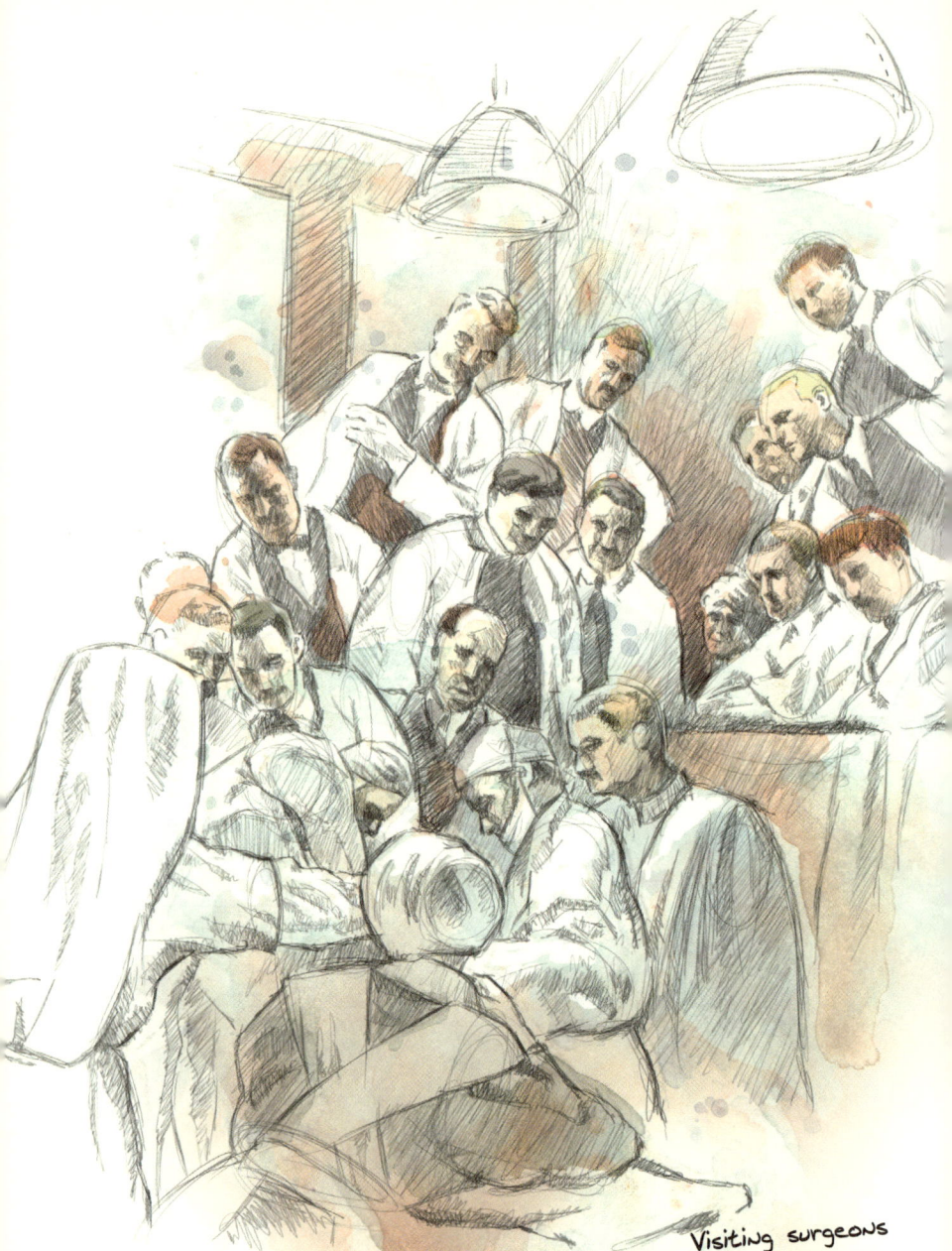

Visiting surgeons filled the observation gallery.

CHAPTER TWO

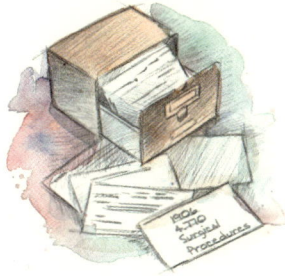

INNOVATION

"We were a green crew and we knew it."

— Dr. Will Mayo

"THE HOSPITAL MUST BE THE BEST AND THE MOST MODERN that means allowed." With these words Dr. W.W. Mayo set his personal standard for building Saint Marys Hospital. To that end he took his older son, Dr. Will, on a tour of Eastern hospitals to study floor plans, lighting arrangements and administrative organization. His younger son, Dr. Charlie, visited hospitals in Europe where he observed new developments in surgical procedures and practice. In consultation with the Sisters, the Mayos pooled their findings and gave the architect instructions "once and twice and thrice" until they got exactly what they wanted.

The Mayo brothers avidly sought innovative ideas and methods. They reserved application, however, to those changes that furthered their primary purpose. Dr. Will put it succinctly: "To get the patient well with as little loss of time as possible: whatever contributes to this end is adopted; whatever does not is eliminated."

In the early years, Dr. Charlie used his mechanical skills to solve hospital problems ... albeit with varying degrees of success. The hospital had no paging system. Dr. Charlie and a neighbor boy installed an electric announcing system. As the story goes, these amateur electricians got some wires crossed. "The bells would start ringing and would not stop." The Sisters carried shears with them as a precaution. If a bell kept on ringing, swish! went the wires. The next morning Dr. Charlie would have to resurrect the whole system again.

The hospital desperately needed an elevator. Good fortune brought an unlikely helper to the door. The Sisters always offered hobos a good meal. One day, a well-traveled hobo described a hydraulic elevator he had seen in Paris. Hearing this, Dr. Charlie and a local machinist dug a 40-foot hole and lowered several sections of pipe into it. When water from the basement reservoir rushed into the pipe, it pushed the elevator upward like a giant syringe.

The hobo described the elevator he saw in Paris.

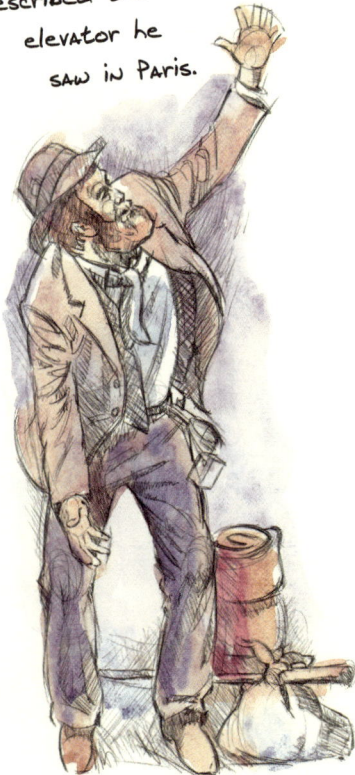

The Mayo brothers kept looking for new ways to improve medicine.

Saint Marys Hospital opened as a new era of surgery began. Infection was a surgeon's greatest nemesis and the reason for the public's fear of hospitals. Even after successful surgical procedures, septic infections invaded patient wounds, causing high fever and, many times, death. In 1867, Scottish surgeon Joseph Lister demonstrated that bacterial microorganisms caused surgical infection and that antisepsis could kill them. Wherever surgeons practiced antisepsis, operations increased in volume and scope. The Mayos incorporated antisepsis in their surgery with astonishing results: of the 1,037 patients admitted in the first two years, the number of deaths was 22, as low as at any time in the hospital's history. Patients went home cured and, in turn, told others about their experience. Such a low mortality rate, which brought recognition for the abilities of the Doctors Mayo, also brought increasing numbers of patients to Saint Marys Hospital.

Fired with ambition to create a surgical center on a level with Eastern hospitals, the Mayos kept abreast of new developments. In Dr. Will's words, "We were a green crew and we knew it." Yet, it was their consuming

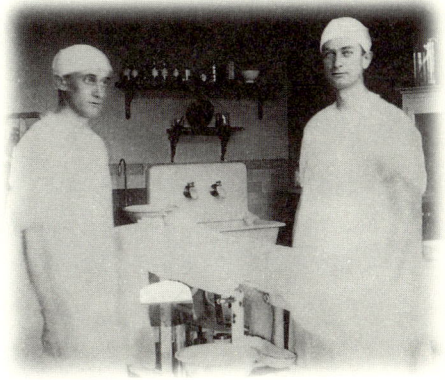

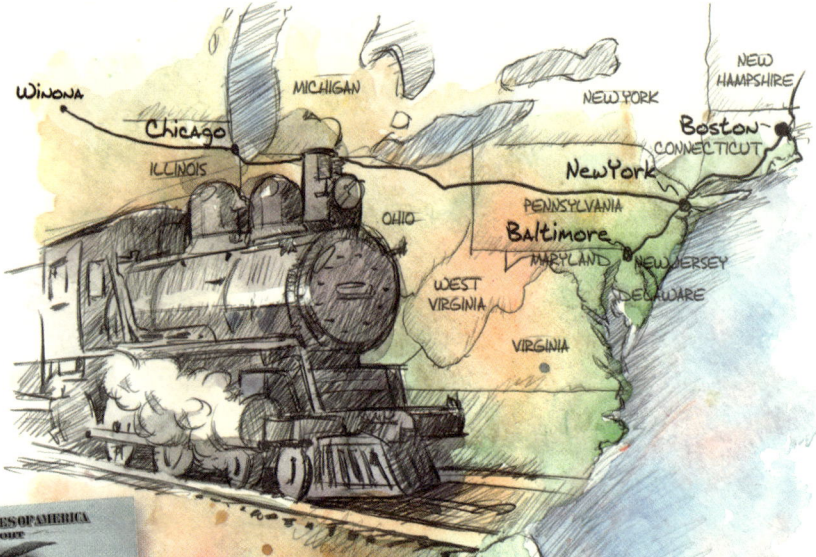

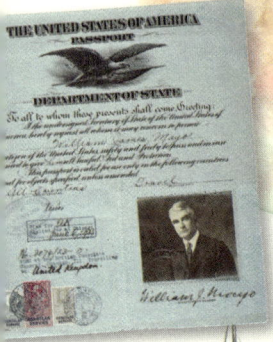

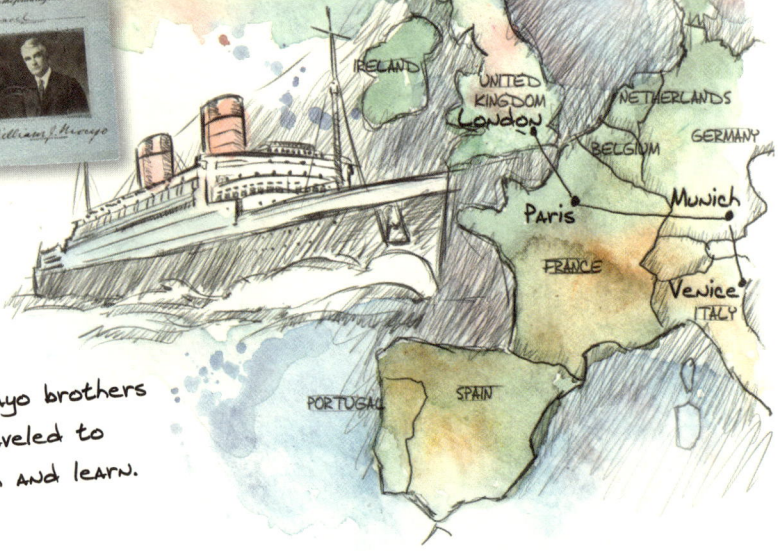

The Mayo brothers traveled to teach and learn.

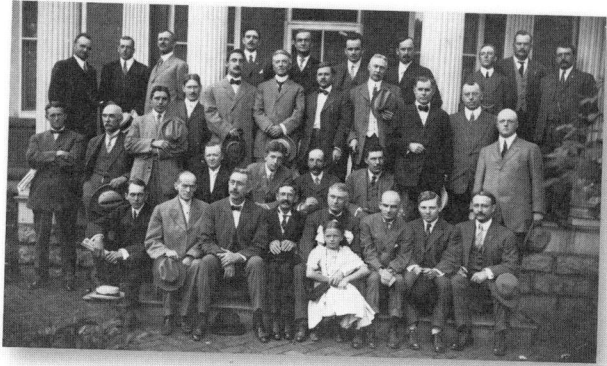

Dr. Will and his daughter, Phoebe, photographed with a group of surgeons visiting Rochester.

desire to overcome inadequacy that helped build the Mayo team of surgeons. One at a time, over several years, they made extended visits to leading surgical centers in Baltimore, Boston, Philadelphia and Chicago to observe the work of selected surgeons. The Mayos were determined to bring back from every trip some specific improvement that could be applied in Rochester, even if it was only a new kind of soap or antiseptic. When one of them returned from a trip, Sister Joseph Dempsey, the superintendent of Saint Marys, would remark, "Now I wonder what new things we will need to do." The Sisters were as committed to improving in their areas of practice as the Mayos were in surgery.

Working in their remote location, far from urban centers and nearby competitors, the Mayos performed some operations by the hundreds, and even by the thousands. Indeed, by 1906 the Mayo surgeons had performed 4,770 operations, more than any hospital in the United States.

Visiting surgeons wore these ribbons when they observed procedures in the operating room.

REPORTER **No.1**
Surgeons' Club

PORTER **No.3**
Surgeons' Club

ORTER **No.4**
Surgeons' Club

PORTER **No.5**
Surgeons' Club

PORTER **No.6**
geons' Club

As the Mayo brothers acquired prominence, large numbers of surgeons, both national and international, came to Rochester. They were fascinated that two unheralded surgeons, native sons of the Midwest, should have developed a center of surgery in an out-of-the-way village. The large number of surgeries daily in many fields permitted demonstration of all the newer surgical procedures in the course of a few days. Visitors could not only witness the technical skills of the Mayos, but could hear them discuss surgical problems in their operating rooms. Their simple, informal remarks reflected the personalities of the Mayos themselves who were frank, unassuming and honest men.

ENDNOTES

Page 12: A firsthand account of the hobo who described an elevator he saw in Paris is covered in a dictated note entitled "Elevator" from Sister Sylvester Burke to Sister Mary Brigh Cassidy, *Saint Marys Hospital Archives.*

Page 15: The Sisters' and the Mayos' dedication to improvement is described in **Whelan, E: *The Sisters' Story: Saint Marys Hospital – Mayo Clinic.* Rochester, Minnesota: Mayo Foundation for Medical Education and Research. Volume One, Second Edition, 2016; p. 81.**

Page 15: Early statistics can be found in the *Annals of Saint Marys Hospital.*

CHECK YOUR COMPASS

INNOVATION

Infuse and energize the organization, enhancing the lives of those we serve, through the creative ideas and unique talents of each employee.

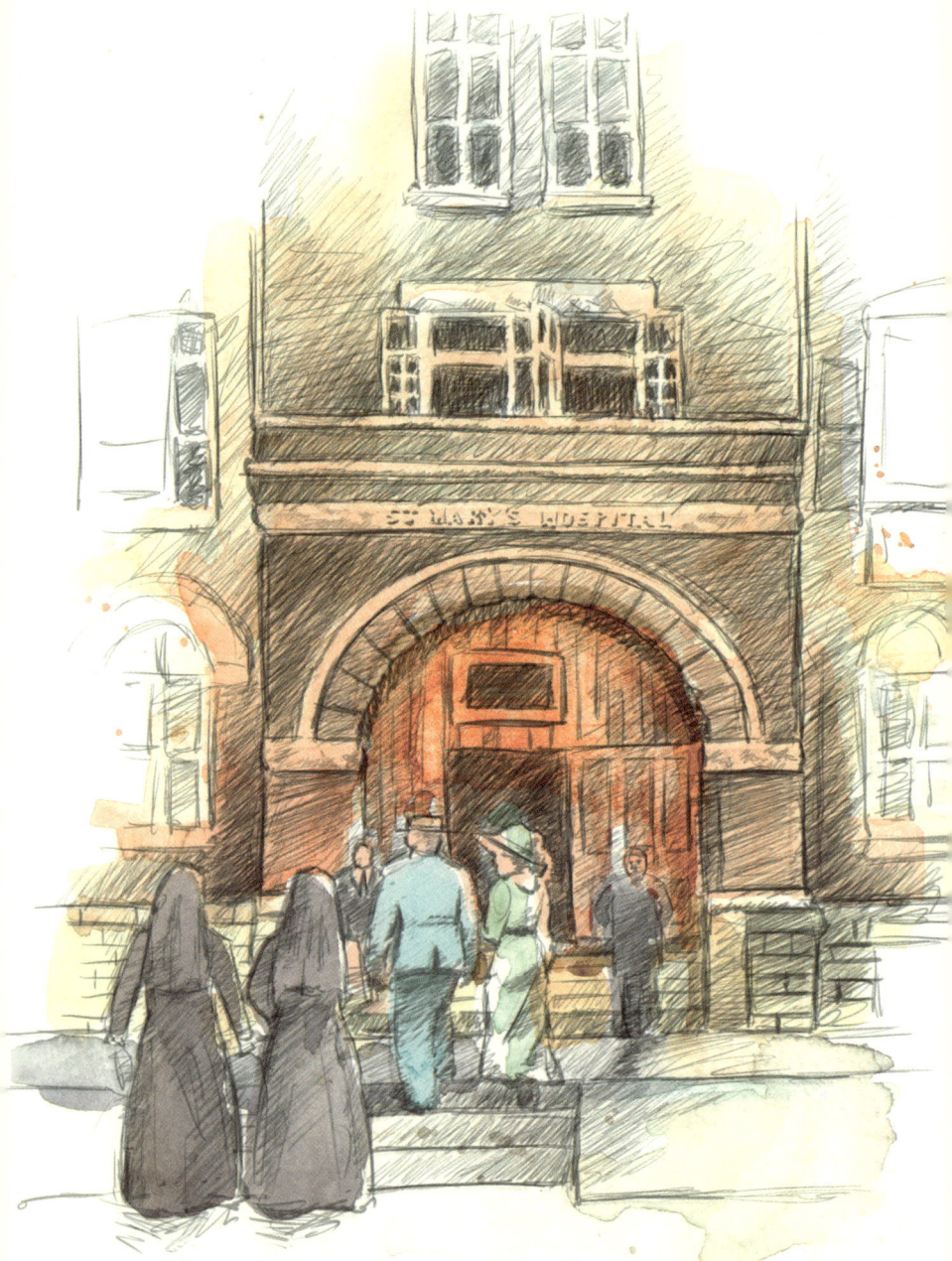

Patients came to Saint Marys
from near and far.

CHAPTER THREE

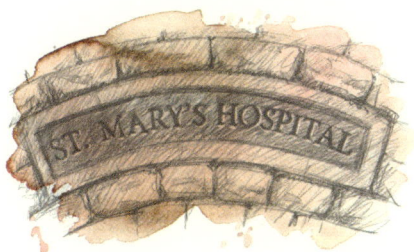

INTEGRITY

"The cause of suffering humanity knows no religion."

— Mother Alfred Moes

THE PARTNERSHIP OF THE YOUNG MAYOS AND THE FRANCISCAN Sisters began tentatively. At first glance, they appeared to have little in common. The Protestant Mayos may have viewed religious life with some admiration, but it was clearly outside their experience. Despite the diversity of backgrounds, the Mayo brothers and the Franciscan Sisters trusted each other's commitment to a common goal, the care of suffering humanity. Such commitment inspired unstinting effort, tapped creative resources and transcended religious differences. They forged a permanent partnership and in the process overcame formidable obstacles. Anti-Catholicism, however, was an obstacle that even high spirits and great resolve could not overcome.

Three years after the hospital opened, the Franciscans and Mayos faced a critical challenge. Saint Marys opened to serve all sick persons regardless of their color, financial resources or professed religion.

Mother Alfred put it clearly: "The cause of suffering humanity knows no religion ..." When Dr. W.W. Mayo, at Mother Alfred's request, tried to organize a staff, he met with evasion and outright refusal. The physicians he approached wanted no part of a venture that was sure to fail because of rising anti-Catholicism.

Between 1860 and 1890 the Catholic population in America tripled and continued to grow. Waves of immigration alarmed native-born Protestants who feared for the country's stability. Nativism centered in the Midwest through the American Protective Association (APA), a secret society, successor to the Know-Nothings and forerunner of the Ku Klux Klan. "Ardent Protestants would have none of an institution that was managed by black-robed nuns and in which there was a chapel set aside for the exercises of popery."

A rival physician, Dr. W. A. Allen, built a competing hospital that offered an alternative to one owned by Catholic Sisters. The new institution,

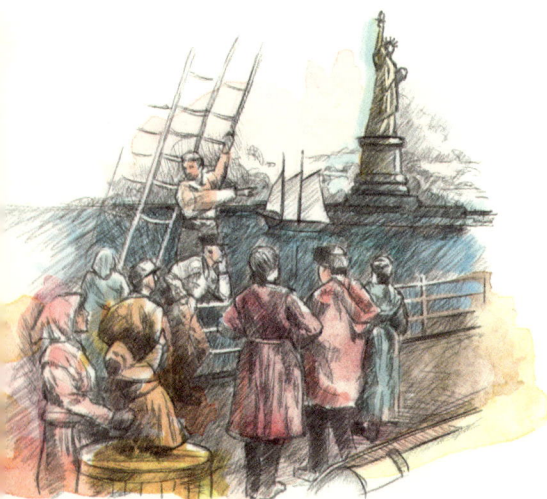

A new life in America.

The Mayo brothers were loyal to each other and to the Sisters.

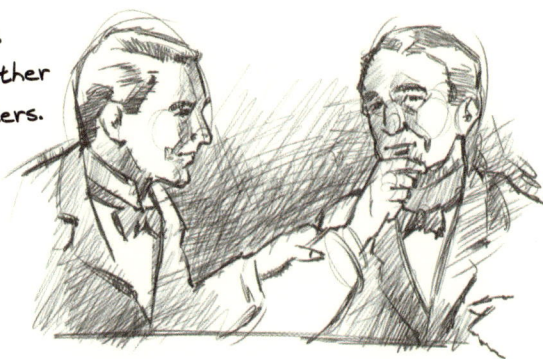

Riverside Hospital, opened for patients in November 1892. Local Protestants pointed to the rival Riverside as an institution that Protestants and patriots could enter "without doing outrage to their convictions by furthering an agency of the hated and alien Catholic Church."

At this juncture, two important members of the Presbyterian Church fell ill and were taken to Riverside Hospital. They called on the Doctors Mayo to attend them. The Mayos faced an important decision. To accept patients at the rival hospital would have disastrous consequences for Saint Marys since most of their patients would then choose the non-Catholic hospital. After deliberating, the Mayos refused to attend patients or to operate in Riverside Hospital. "To divert a share of their practice to another hospital seemed wrong," writes their biographer, "a poor return for loyalty and confidence. Moreover, the Mayos felt a strong moral

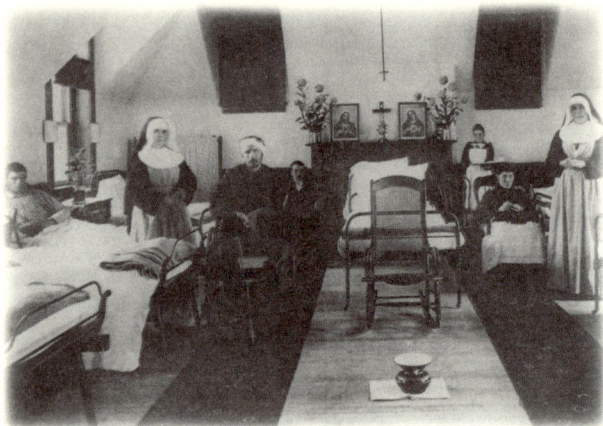

Compassion and
care for
every patient.

obligation to the Sisters of St. Francis. And, finally, the Mayos were not men inclined to knuckle under to the public clamor or the pressure of opposition."

As anticipated, their decision brought highly emotional censure and criticism from a segment of the Protestant community. In the midst of these contentious times, the Mayos quietly focused on their practice and cared for patients. When critics attacked them and waited for a response, they chose to ignore the abuse and appeared unperturbed.

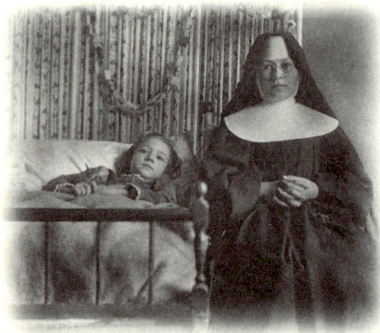

Riverside Hospital was in operation for over two years when Dr. Allen made a startling announcement. For unknown reasons, "at the peak of prosperity and popularity," he was leaving his practice and moving to St. Paul. Shortly after he left, the hospital closed and sold its beds and other movables to Saint Marys.

Presumably, this was an extraordinarily difficult time for the Sisters, particularly since they were powerless to do anything about pervasive anti-Catholicism. They wanted their institution to succeed, but in truth, they believed the success of the hospital was not up to them; it was in God's hands. And so, as was their custom in times of difficulty and decision, they fasted and prayed that God would bless the work of their hands.

The strident competition over Riverside Hospital cemented the relationship between the Doctors Mayo and the Sisters at Saint Marys. Despite inexperience, hardship and hostility, they had learned to depend upon each other. The Sisters would never forget how the doctors endured public abuse with steadfast courage on their behalf. The Mayos' unswerving loyalty had almost certainly saved the hospital. The Mayos, forced by circumstances, found they could furnish all the patients needed for the

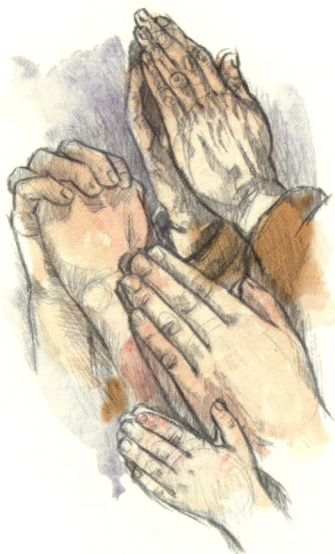

The Sisters prayed that God would bless the work of their hands.

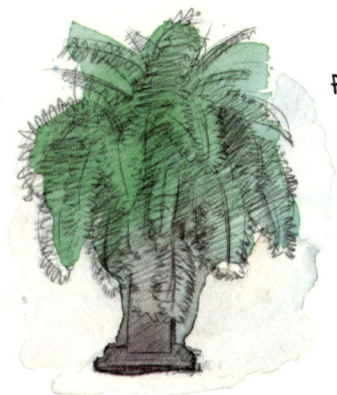

Plants & flowers made the hospital feel like home.

hospital. In turn, the Sisters demonstrated they could provide all the doctors needed in a hospital and nursing care. Each made the decision to rely solely on the other. The Mayos' decision centralized their surgical practice and became a primary factor in their phenomenal success. The Sisters' decision moved Saint Marys Hospital beyond perceived parochial boundaries and into the mainstream of America.

ENDNOTES

Pages 20-24: The story of Riverside Hospital is included in **Clapesattle, pp. 264-267**, and **Whelan, Volume One, pp. 71-73**. In addition, the *Annals of Saint Marys Hospital*, 1892, provides contemporary information.

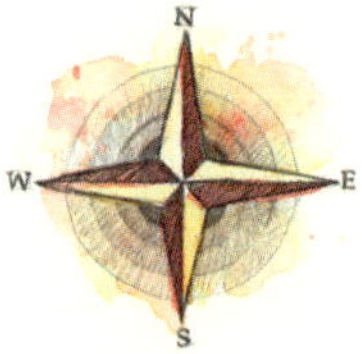

CHECK YOUR COMPASS

INTEGRITY

Adhere to the highest standards of professionalism, ethics and personal responsibility, worthy of the trust our patients place in us.

_____

_____

_____

_____

_____

_____

_____

_____

_____

_____

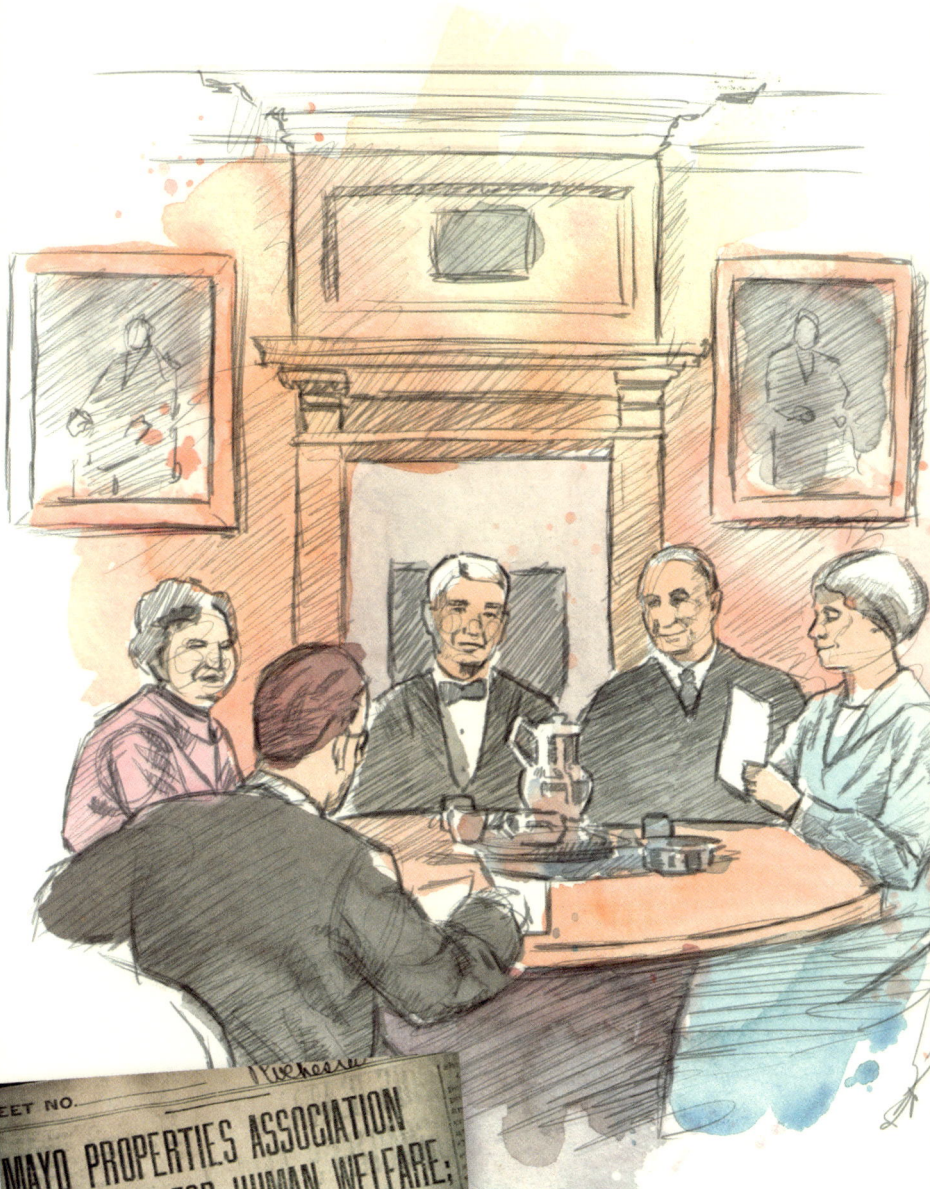

MAYO PROPERTIES ASSOCIATION
ORGANIZED FOR HUMAN WELFARE;
NO CAPITAL STOCK; ALL CLINIC
PROPERTIES IN MAYOS' GIFT

A transformative gift.

CHAPTER FOUR

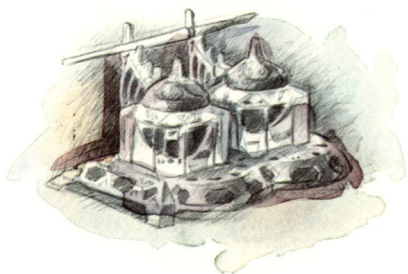

STEWARDSHIP

"... contributions to the general good of humanity."

— Deed of Gift

IN A SINGULAR ACT OF RENUNCIATION AND DEDICATION, THE MAYO brothers took a series of steps in the years surrounding World War I that would alleviate sickness and suffering for future generations of patients. By transforming Mayo Clinic from a private partnership into a not-for-profit organization, they "made the medical experience of past generations available for the coming one." In the words of Dr. Will, "Each new generation shall not have to work out its problems independently, but may begin where its predecessors left off." The brothers solidified their commitment by donating the majority of their life savings, as well as all the physical properties and assets of Mayo Clinic. At the time, the total value of their generosity was more than $10 million; the equivalent sum today would be many times greater.

According to the Deed of Gift signed by both brothers and their wives, along with other related documents, the Mayos, their partners and all future Mayo Clinic personnel would receive a salary and not profit personally from the proceeds of the practice. All proceeds beyond operating expenses would be contributed to education, research and patient care. This was a bold step and ensured that Mayo would survive beyond its founders' retirements and deaths. From this initiative Mayo Clinic emerged as a distinct institution and a new model of private group practice.

The decision grew out of the Mayo brothers' shared surgical practice that began 30 years earlier. At first the brothers operated together because they found their combined technical skills produced the best results. Each took turns serving as the other's first assistant. The brothers discussed every feature of their operations and pooled knowledge and ingenuity to meet a crisis when it came. Together, they faced and fought through problems, shouldered responsibilities and won successes. In the process they forged a bond of mutual love and admiration, "a bond so strong that nothing could ever break it."

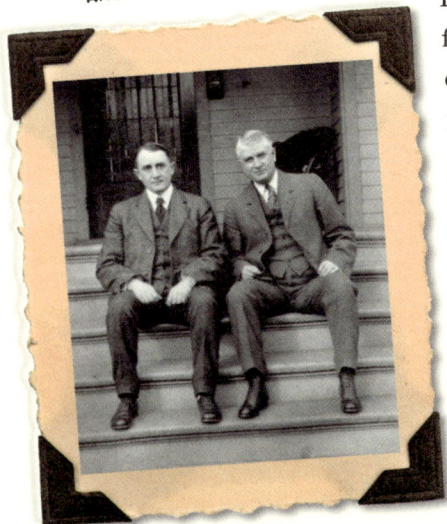

"My brother and I"

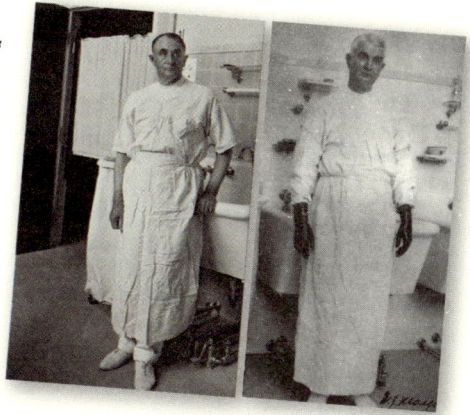

Surgeons and humanitarian leaders.

Despite outward differences, their personal respect and commitment to each other was unshakable. When talking about themselves, they rarely used "I" or "me," but preferred to say, "my brother and I." A colleague in later years remarked, "Your great success was not as surgeons. It was as brothers; there has never been anything like it."

The Mayo brothers' unqualified trust in each other extended to their finances. Indeed, they shared the same checkbook. Ten years into their surgical practice, when Dr. Will was 33 and Dr. Charlie 29, the brothers took stock of their finances. Over the course of several discussions, they agreed that half of their earnings was sufficient for themselves and their families. The remaining funds, in their words, "should be returned to the people from whom it came in a way that would do them the greatest benefit." The brothers made a solemn vow to set aside half of their income that year and as much each year thereafter as they could. "They would invest it and increase it to the best of their ability, and someday they would find a way to return it to the people."

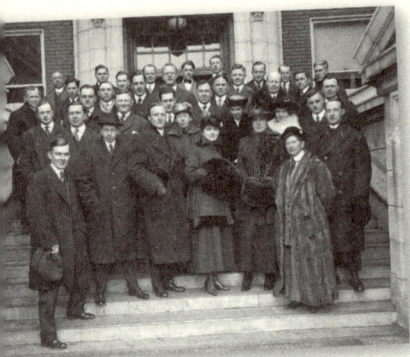

Young doctors came to study at Mayo Clinic.

By 1917, the brothers' plans moved toward fruition, "but not without a struggle." The brothers transferred funds to the University of Minnesota in order to support advanced specialty training for physicians and scientists using Mayo Clinic facilities and staff in Rochester. Affiliated with the university, their moneys would help establish "the first American graduate school in clinical medicine."

News of the proposed affiliation with the university infuriated many Minnesota doctors. For some, their motive was a long-standing fear and jealousy of the Mayos' success. Others held valid criticisms of the plan as it stood. "None of those elements, however," writes biographer Helen Clapesattle, "can account for the personal spite and malice, the disgraceful misrepresentation." Opponents lobbied the Minnesota legislature to pass a bill against the affiliation. When a public hearing was announced, friends and colleagues urged Dr. Will to speak to the legislative assembly. He hesitated, then responded, "I'm a good soldier. If you gentlemen think it's necessary, I'll do it."

The chamber was crowded the night of the hearing. People hushed as Dr. Mayo began to speak. He talked without notes, earnestly, simply, colloquially. "Every man has some inspiration; with my brother and I, it came from our father. He taught us that any man who has physical strength, intellectual capacity or unusual opportunity holds such endowments in trust, to do with them for others in proportion to his gifts." His voice rose. "Now let's call a spade a spade. This money belongs to the people and I don't care two raps whether the medical profession of the state likes the way this money has been offered for use or not. It wasn't their money." Lowering his tone, Dr. Will recalled the words of Abraham Lincoln, "... that these dead shall not have died in vain." He said this line "explains why we want to do this thing. ... What better could we do than take young men and help them to become proficient in the profession so as to prevent needless deaths?" The bill failed.

The ultimate success of Mayo Clinic, "past, present and future, must be measured largely by its contributions to the general good of humanity." Inspired by their founders' pledge in 1919, future generations at Mayo Clinic went on to greater levels of accomplishment and service.

Dr. Will admired Abraham Lincoln.

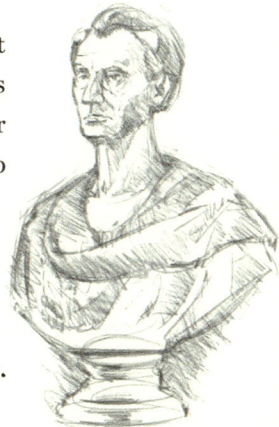

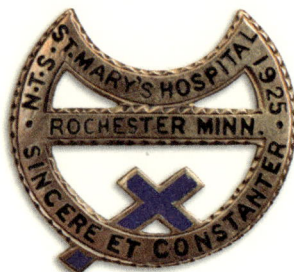

Saint Marys School of Nursing was nationally recognized for excellence.

ENDNOTES

Page 27:   The Mayo family's altruistic philosophy is described in **Beck, CS:** *Teamwork at Mayo Clinic.* **Rochester, Minnesota: Mayo Foundation for Medical Education and Research, 2014, p. 11.**

Page 28:   The evolution of the Mayo brothers' thinking in establishing the not-for-profit organization is described in **Hartzell, J:** *I Started All This – The Life of Dr. William Worrall Mayo.* **Greenville, South Carolina: Arvi Books, 2004, p. 158.**

Pages 30-31: The "Lost Oration," as Dr. Will's informal speech to the Minnesota Legislature was called, is described and quoted in **Willius, F:** *Aphorisms.* **Rochester, Minnesota: Mayo Foundation for Medical Education and Research, 1990, pp. 85-92.**

Page 31:   **Mayo Clinic Archives** contain the ***Deed of Gift from William J. Mayo and Charles H. Mayo to Mayo Properties Association, October 8, 1919.*** The deed's purpose in serving "the general good of humanity" is stated on **page 3.**

CHECK YOUR COMPASS

STEWARDSHIP

Sustain and reinvest in our mission and extended communities by wisely managing our human, natural and material resources.

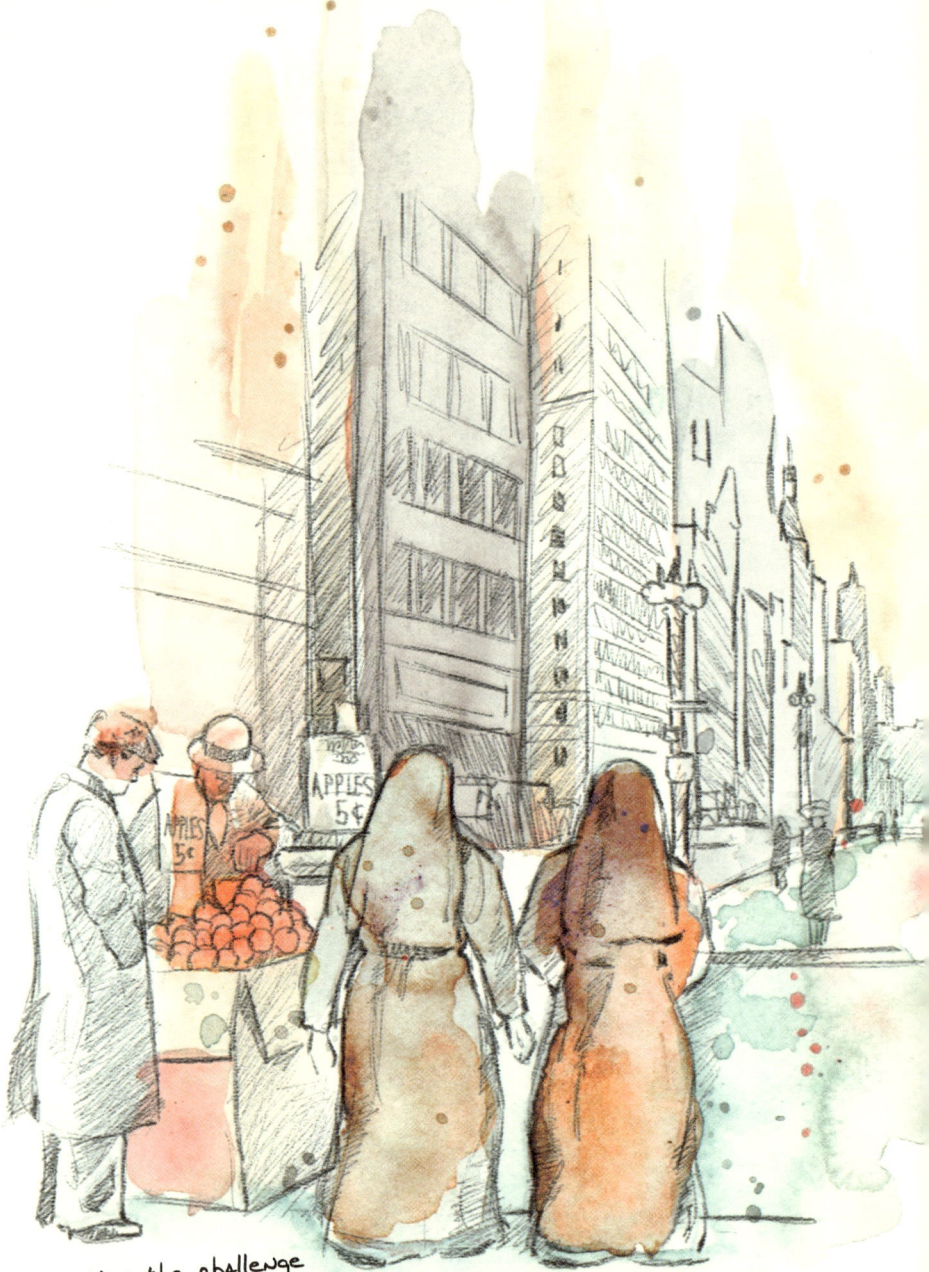

Meeting the challenge
of the Great Depression.

CHAPTER FIVE

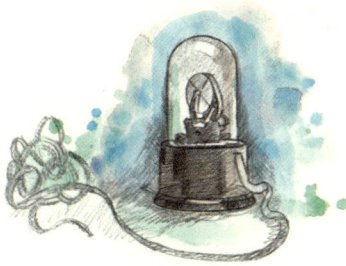

TEAMWORK

"We were our own brokers ... We never missed our prayers."

— Sister Adele O'Neil

A SUCCESSFUL TEAM ENLISTS THE RIGHT PARTNERS, EVEN WHEN THEY are unlikely collaborators. In the middle of the Great Depression, Sister Adele O'Neil, an intrepid little Franciscan in Rochester, Minnesota, stepped forward to help save her congregation from bankruptcy.

The Great Depression had drastic consequences for Saint Marys Hospital and the Rochester Franciscan congregation. Large debts for an extensive building project in the 1920s came due in the early 1930s. In 1933, the Sisters elected a new mother superior, Mother Aquinas Norton, known for her "organizational ability and financial genius." On her first day in office, the sheriff came to Mother Aquinas' door to inform her that she was liable for a debt of $5 million owed to 5,000 note holders. Unknown to her, the congregation's business agent in Chicago, charged with the debt repayment, had absconded with $350,000 of the Sisters' money.

Mother Aquinas' first order of business was to extricate the congregation from threatened bankruptcy. She immediately appointed Sister Adele O'Neil as congregational treasurer. Young, lively and petite, Sister Adele possessed disarming financial expertise and dogged determination. Like Mother Aquinas, she learned about finance from working with her family's business before entering the congregation.

Mother Aquinas asked the Bishop of Winona, Minnesota, Francis M. Kelly, and his advisors to meet about the financial crisis. To their surprise, the diminutive Sister Adele spoke up and suggested that she serve as broker rather than pay a large commission to a hired agent. Given the desperate situation, they agreed. Later, Sister Adele told the astonishing story of how she repaid the note holders and "no one lost a dollar of principal."

The Sisters took a train to Chicago to meet with their creditors.

Sister Adele chose Sister Rita Rishavy, the business officer of Saint Marys Hospital, as her assistant. With 80 percent of their creditors in Chicago, Sister Adele sought assistance from a large Chicago bank. As she put it, "We made friends with the Continental Bank of Chicago and

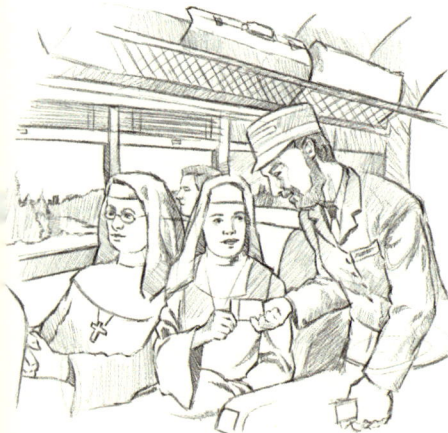

Continental Bank,
Chicago, c. 1933.

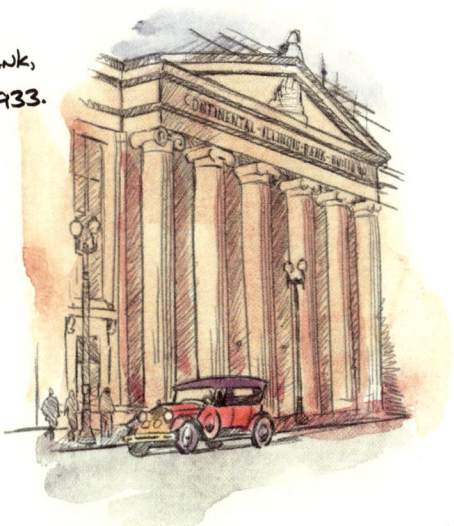

found the vice president very helpful." He gave them regular use of a conference room with telephone and typewriter. The room opened on the office of the bank's legal officer, who offered his services as needed. Thus began the financial odyssey of Sister Adele and Sister Rita to and from Chicago, twice weekly, over the next several months.

The Chicago and North Western Railroad, which served Rochester, gave free passes to religious Sisters. Since there was no day train, the Sisters traveled at night. Upon arrival in Chicago, they stopped at a downtown church for Mass, then went to the Continental Bank. They worked the full day, asking creditors to renew their notes at a lower percentage. "Any one of them could have thrown us into bankruptcy," Sister Adele reflected, "but they gladly agreed in order to save their principal." Returning to Rochester, the Sisters went directly to the motherhouse and wrote to the creditors, often until midnight, without benefit of any office machines but a manual typewriter. After a day, sometimes two, they went back to Chicago and repeated the

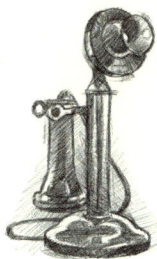

"We were our
own brokers ...
we never missed
our prayers."

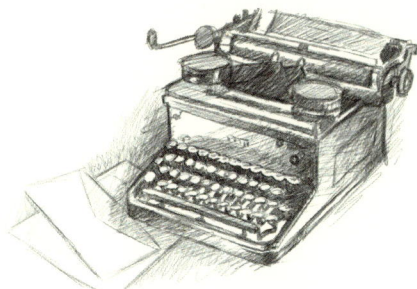

process. "Through it all," Sister Adele was quick to say, "we never missed our prayers."

Six years later, when Saint Marys Hospital needed $8 million to build a medical wing, Sister Adele again approached the Continental Bank of Chicago. The bank, she recalled with a smile, "made the loan without a commitment fee." Next, Sister Adele contacted many of the same creditors who had helped save the congregation from bankruptcy. "Almost 100 percent were willing to reinvest." Her eyes sparkled. "From then on, we were our own brokers."

ENDNOTES

Pages 35-36:   Description by Mother Aquinas Norton of the sheriff at her door and subsequent meeting with Bishop Francis Kelly are included in an interview with Sister Bibiana Lewis, May 10, 2001. *Archives of the Sisters of St. Francis, Assisi Heights, Rochester, Minnesota.*

Pages 36-39:   The financial odyssey of Sister Adele O'Neil and Sister Rita Rishavy is described in a taped interview with Sister Adele by Sister Patricia Leon, February 29, 1980. *Archives of the Sisters of St. Francis, Assisi Heights, Rochester, Minnesota.*

CHECK YOUR COMPASS

TEAMWORK

Value the contributions of all, blending the skills of individual staff members in unsurpassed collaboration.

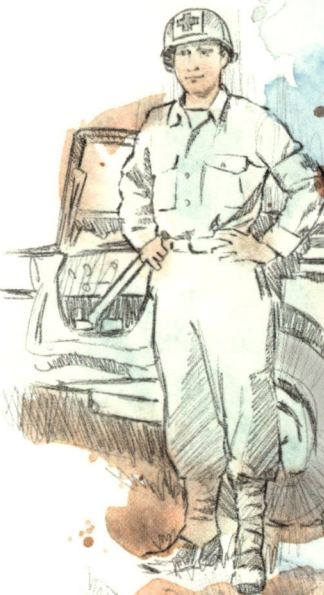

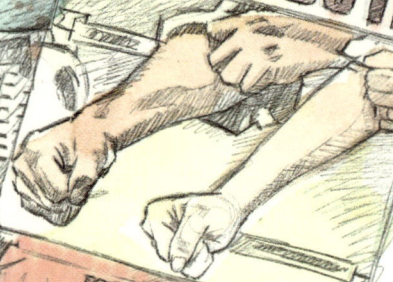

TOGETHER WE CAN DO IT!

KEEP 'EM FIR...

Serving on the battlefield and the home front.

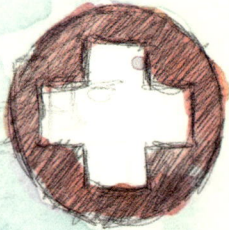

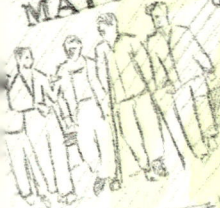

MAYO CLINIC in New Guinea

DECEMBER 7, 1941

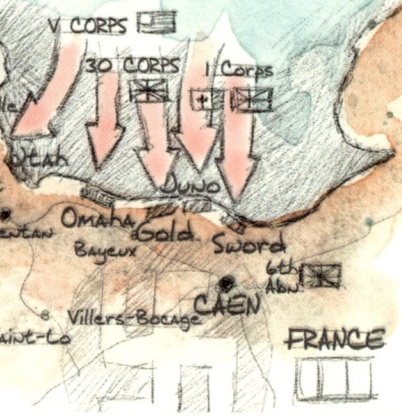

VII CORPS

V CORPS

30 CORPS | CORPS

Cherbourg

Quineville

82nd Abn

101st Abn

Carentan

Utah

Omaha

Bayeux

Juno

Gold

Sword

6th Abn

Saint-Lô

Villers-Bocage

CAEN

FRANCE

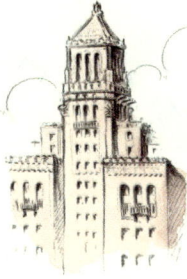

CHAPTER SIX

HEALING

"I have never forgotten her kindness and concern."

— Sumiko Ito, R.N.

DURING WORLD WAR II THE MAYO CLINIC AND SAINT MARYS HOSPITAL staff served wounded military personnel overseas and ill patients in Rochester with selfless heroism. Almost 300 Mayo physicians volunteered for the armed forces. In Rochester, their colleagues worked round-the-clock caring for record numbers of patients. Harry Harwick, Mayo's chief administrator, described the war years. "The Clinic contributed heavily in manpower, perhaps a third of our consultants, including ranking members in many specialties, a good third of our Fellows and, it sometimes seemed, almost every able-bodied man of military age in the nonmedical sections. With this depleted staff, we were faced with registrations that reached record numbers." Deferring their retirements, many senior physicians "took on work loads more suitable to men half their age, and handled them superbly."

41

Like his colleagues, surgeon O. T. Clagett, M.D., "carried the extra burden with a spirit that has never been excelled in the history of the Clinic." He recalled, "I believe my longest surgical list in one day was 23 major operations." "Lists of 15 to 20 operations daily were almost routine. I remember one day I had a list of 19 operations. A visitor in the gallery spoke to me in the course of the day and said, 'I am the medical officer who examined you at Fort Snelling and turned you down as unfit for active military service. I think I made a hell of a mistake.'"

At Saint Marys Hospital, Sisters and staff met wartime shortages with equal spirit. A sentence in the hospital newsletter captured their resolve. "We must learn the true meaning of sacrifice, of more work, faster work and of one more job." Prayer was an essential part of the Sisters' day. Whether in chapel or catching a minute on the floors, they prayed for the armed forces and those who bore the burdens of war at home. "Healing in body and spirit" was their prayer and their practical means of support to help the displaced persons of Japanese descent living on the West Coast. Feared as enemy

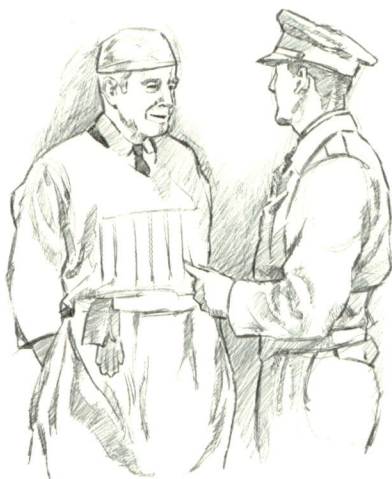

"Lists of 15 to 20 operations a day were almost routine."

agents, 120,000 Japanese-Americans were forcibly re-moved from their homes, jobs and schools to live in "war re-location camps." Following the Japanese attack on Pearl Harbor, armed soldiers herded adults and children into tar-paper barracks without running water and adequate heat.

The plight of Japanese-American nursing students troubled Sister Antonia Rostomily, director of Saint Marys School of Nursing. A formidable teacher and disciplinarian, Sister Antonia was a woman of good heart and common sense. Aware that many nursing schools would not accept Japanese-American students, she believed Saint Marys Hospital with its experience in serving international patients would be a desirable setting. With strong support from hospital administration, the nursing school faculty and student body, her proposal went forward. The admissions committee selected 15 Japanese-American applicants, "for their scholastic ability, educational, and social background."

For the young Japanese-American nursing students, the welcome opportunity came at a wrenching cost. They

Japanese-Americans were sent to detention camps.

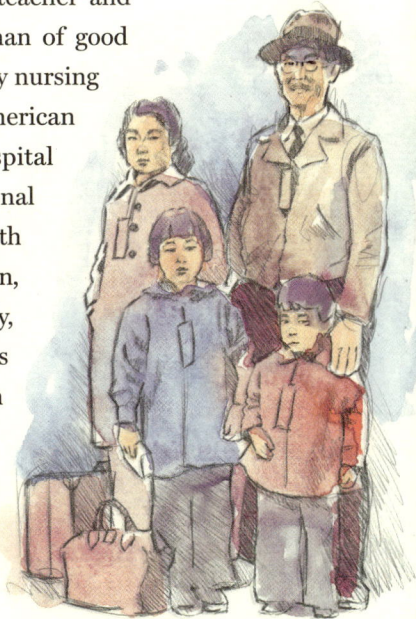

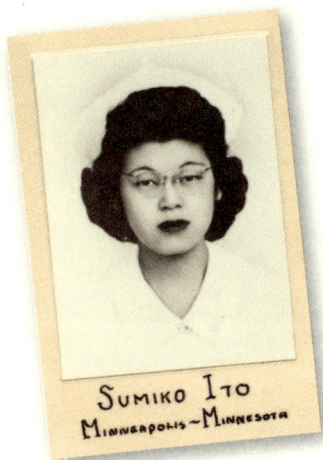

Sumiko Ito
Minneapolis~Minnesota

Sumiko Ito
learned
nursing skills at
Saint Marys
Hospital.

left beloved parents and siblings imprisoned in primitive barracks, surrounded by armed guards and barbed wire. It is difficult to imagine their thoughts as they boarded trains that took them to Rochester, a 2,000-mile journey into a Minnesota winter and an unknown future.

Fifty years later, in 1994, one of the students, Sumiko Ito, wrote a letter to the nursing school's alumni office. She shared a life-changing experience that happened early in her student days. "It was with a thankful heart and a fierce determination to succeed that I entered my probationary period," she recalled. "Toward the end of my probation, a bunch of us were invited to a get-together at a friend's house. Time got away from us. We feared we would miss our curfew and ran all the way back to the nurses' home." They missed the curfew by minutes. The next morning a note on the bulletin board summoned the offenders to Sister Antonia's office.

"With great trepidation," Sumiko wrote, "I entered her door. To my vast astonishment, Sister Antonia did not admonish or discipline us. Instead, she said she wanted to talk with us. Knowing we were undergoing many adjustments and were subject to racial intolerance, she asked how we were doing and if everyone was treating us well. She used this episode just to talk to us. I have never forgotten her kindness and concern."

Sister Antonia and many of the Sisters who prayed for Japanese-Americans did not live to read Sumiko's letter. Yet surely long before, they were confident that their prayers brought healing and solace for Sumiko and her people.

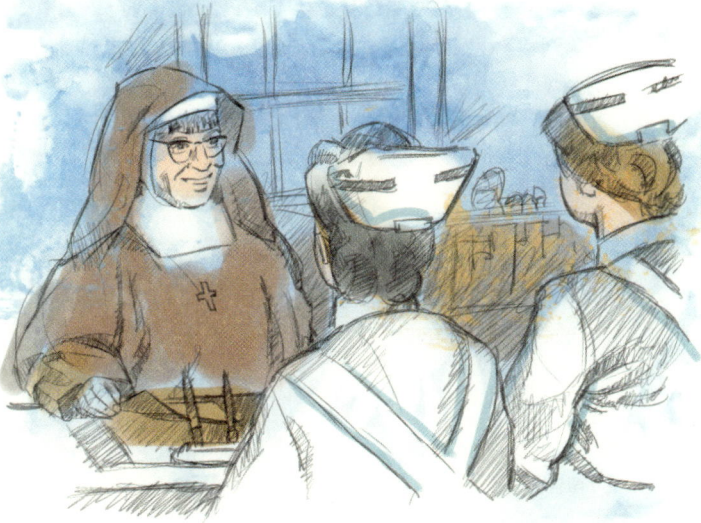

"I have never forgotten Sister Antonia's kindness and concern."

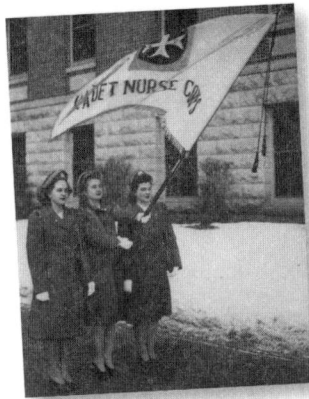

Cadet Nurses trained at Saint Marys during World War II.

ENDNOTES

Page 41:   Harwick, HJ: *Forty-Four Years with the Mayo Clinic*. Rochester, Minnesota: Whiting Press, 1957, p. 33.

Page 42:   The statement "carried the extra burden with a spirit that has never been excelled in the history of the Clinic" comes from Donald C. Balfour, M.D., and is found in the *Balfour Papers,* Mayo Clinic Archives, Rochester, Minnesota.

Page 42:   The vignette about Dr. Clagett is included in Johnson, V: *Mayo Clinic – Its Growth and Progress*. Bloomington, Minnesota: Voyageur Press, 1984, p. 37.

Page 42:   "We must learn the true meaning of sacrifice …" is found in *Saint Marys Hospital Bulletin,* Vol. 1, No. 1, May 1942, p. 3.

Pages 43-44:   "Relocation of American College Students: Acceptance of a Change" is described in Provinse, JH: *Higher Education* 1 (8): 1-4, April 16, 1945.

Page 43:   Information about admitting students to Saint Marys is found in the entry "American-Japanese Students," *Annals of Saint Marys Hospital,* 1943. Americans of Japanese ancestry were hired for several positions at Saint Marys Hospital, including nursing instructor, night supervisor, dietitian, head nurse and secretary for the school of nursing.

Pages 44-45:   The story of Sumiko Ito is recounted in Wentzel, VS: *Sincere et Constanter: 1906-1970 – The Story of Saint Marys School of Nursing.* Rochester, Minnesota: Mayo Foundation for Medical Education and Research, 2006, p. 224.

CHECK YOUR COMPASS

HEALING

Inspire hope and nurture the well-being of the whole person, respecting physical, emotional and spiritual needs.

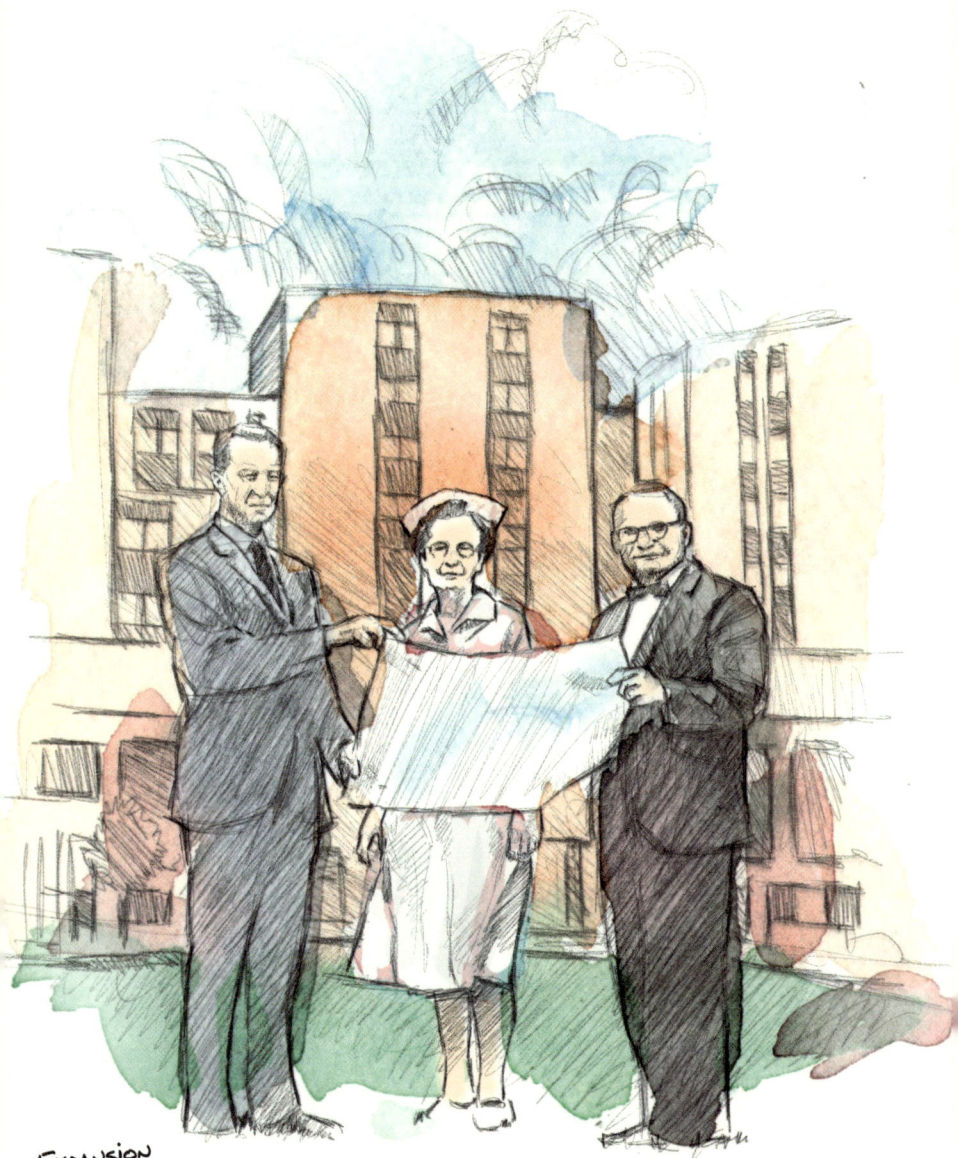

Expansion
in the
post-war era.

CHAPTER SEVEN

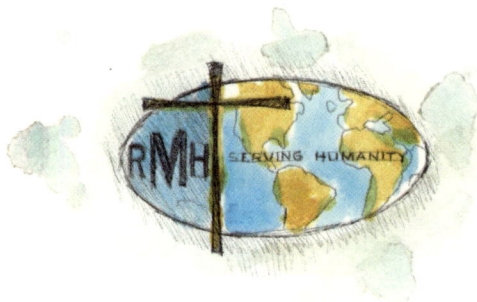

EXCELLENCE

"Do all the good you can ..."

— John Wesley

THE END OF WORLD WAR II HELD GREAT PROMISE. PATIENTS ARRIVED in record numbers. Plans took shape for an extensive new facility: the Mayo Building. Saint Marys Hospital prepared for an increased workload. "Only the downtown hospitals ... flawed the hopeful Rochester medical center picture."

"Downtown" hospital care has a story that is distinct from and complementary to the relationship between Saint Marys and Mayo Clinic. Starting in the early 1900s, Saint Marys could not meet all demands, even with frequent expansion. In addition, patients needed a place to recover after surgery and their families needed lodging.

Rochester businessman John Kahler stepped forward. In 1907, he opened a remodeled house near the Mayos' office. A newspaper reported: "The institution has the novel aspect of being a home, a hospital, a sanitarium and an infirmary, all in one."

For the next 47 years, the Kahler Corporation developed a network of hotels and hospitals, along with other amenities, to serve patients and visitors. At the dedication of the Kahler Hotel in 1921, Dr. William J. Mayo praised John Kahler: "He had the vision, the ability, to see and think and act. He has made possible the Clinic expansion."

With changes in medical technology and economics after World War II, however, the Kahler Corporation turned exclusively to hospitality. The search began for a new model of downtown hospital care.

The Kahler Hotel included hospital facilities.

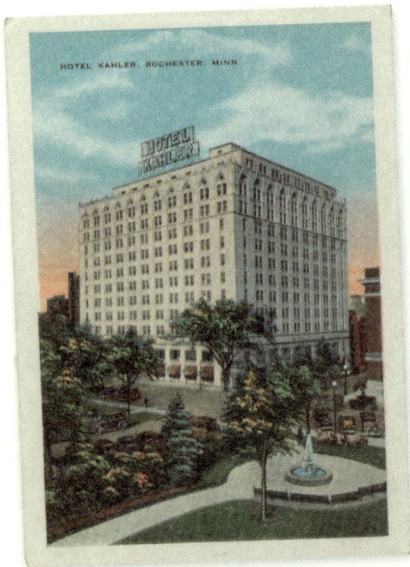

On January 1, 1954, Rochester Methodist Hospital came into being. Like Saint Marys, it was a not-for-profit organization founded by faith-based activists who worked with Mayo physicians. Harry Blackmun, J.D., Mayo Clinic attorney, future justice of the United States Supreme Court and a prominent Methodist, wrote the articles of incorporation.

Unlike Saint Marys, the new hospital was not part of a church hierarchy. It was a stand-alone initia-

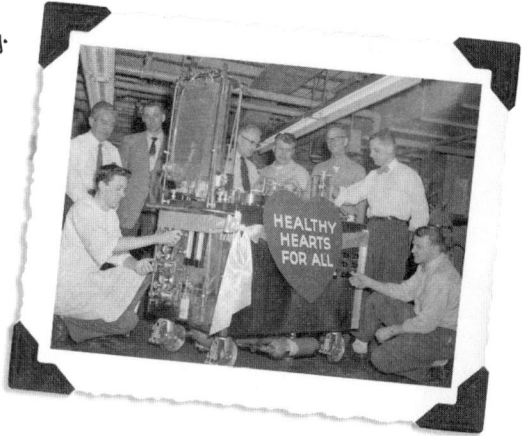

Early days of open-heart surgery.

tive, which compelled innovation. For a dozen years, the staff worked in Kahler facilities constructed decades before. But from the start, they were committed to developing the best methods. Later generations would talk about "Six Sigma" and "Quality Planning." For Rochester Methodist Hospital, the mantra was "Dedicated to Excellence."

In 1955, the hospital earned global acclaim when John Kirklin, M.D., pioneered open-heart surgery with a heart-lung bypass machine. The pharmacy created the unit dose of dispensing medication, setting a new standard for the medical profession. Recognizing the unique ministry of hospital chaplains, Rochester Methodist established a nationally renowned training program for clergy.

Befitting its name, Rochester Methodist Hospital engaged the community. It started a community-based board of directors and auxiliary, later adopted by Saint Marys. While Mayo Clinic and Saint Marys passively accepted gifts, most often for charity care, Rochester Methodist took a proactive approach: setting a vision,

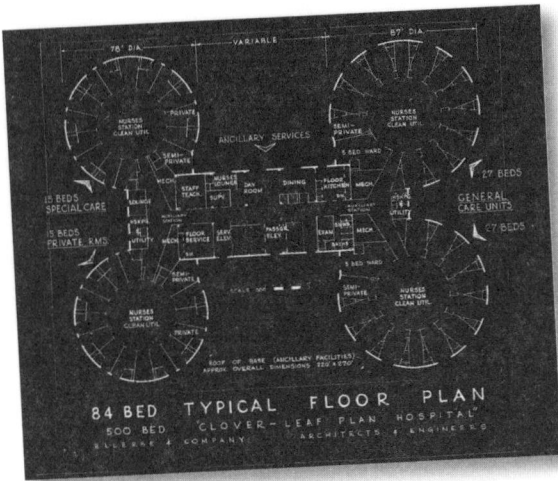

84 BED TYPICAL FLOOR PLAN
500 BED 'CLOVER-LEAF PLAN HOSPITAL'
ELLERBE & COMPANY   ARCHITECTS & ENGINEERS

The radial nursing unit at Rochester Methodist Hospital was a major innovation.

stating a case and seeking support, which defines philanthropy at Mayo Clinic today.

Rochester Methodist also pioneered the respectful way that new management works with established employees ... a spirit that proved essential many times over in the coming years. Rochester Methodist set a bold new path, but welcomed the skills and dedication of former Kahler staff. The revitalized Methodist-Kahler School of Nursing looked ahead while honoring roots of nursing education that went back to 1918.

In 1957, leaders began studying the concept of a radial nursing unit, with a central desk encircled by patient rooms. A prototype nicknamed "the silo" proved its effectiveness. The radial unit became a highlight of the hospital's new building, which opened in 1966, and inspired architects for years to come.

But with progress came sacrifice. Ironically, studies showed the best location for the new building was the site of First Methodist Church, the very congregation that was most deeply involved with the hospital. The congregation gave up its home for a state-of-the-art medical facility and resettled across town as Christ United Methodist Church.

More than 10,000 people thronged to the open house for Rochester Methodist Hospital. Its wide doors opened a new era ... programs in nutrition education ... car seats to give newborn babies a safe ride home ... "Come and See" activities to welcome school children ... the Life Run, an early effort to promote fitness ... the first FDA-approved artificial hip joint ... and Charter House, a new concept in retirement living.

Like Saint Marys, with its Franciscan tradition, Rochester Methodist Hospital was open to people from all walks of life. It took root and flourished with the values of John Wesley, the founder of Methodism, who said: "Do all the good you can, by all the means you can, in all the places you can, at all the times you can, to all the souls you can, for as long as you ever can."

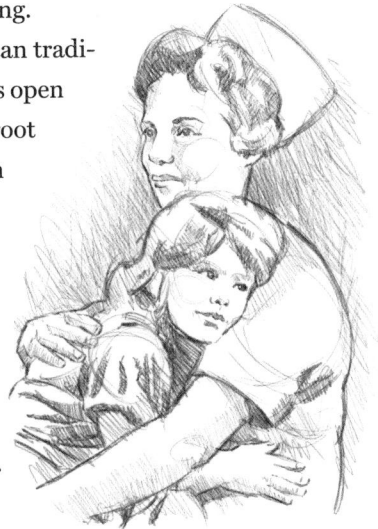

The staff at Rochester Methodist Hospital combined technical skills and compassionate care.

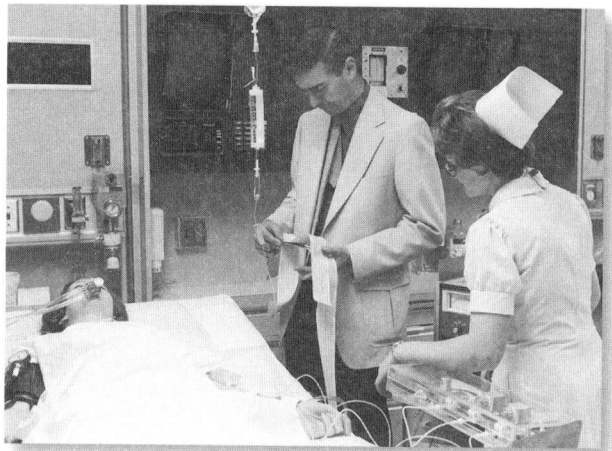

Computers changed the practice of medicine in the 1960s.

ENDNOTES

Page 49:   "Only the downtown hospitals ..." is found in Holmes, W: *Dedicated to Excellence – The Rochester Methodist Hospital Story.* Rochester, Minnesota: Privately printed, 1984; revised, 1987, p. 44.

Page 49:   The 1907 newspaper article is quoted in Holmes, p. 41.

Page 50:   Dr. Will Mayo's speech praising John Kahler at the 1921 dedication of the Kahler Hotel is quoted in *The Kahler Grand Hotel.* Privately printed, no date, p. 1.

Pages 51-53: Milestone accomplishments of Rochester Methodist Hospital are featured in text, artifacts and film in the exhibit, *Dedicated to Excellence: Rochester Methodist Hospital.* Lobby of the George M. Eisenberg Building, Methodist Campus of Mayo Clinic Hospital — Rochester, Rochester, Minnesota.

Page 53:   "Do all the good you can ..." is a saying widely attributed to John Wesley, founder of Methodism, in many print and online sources; wording varies ("souls" vs. "people," etc.).

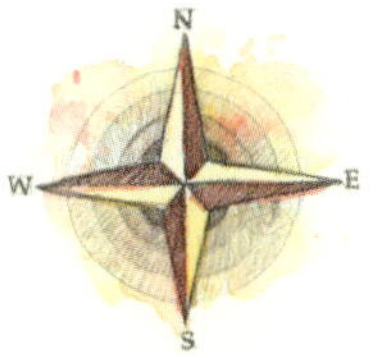

CHECK YOUR COMPASS

EXCELLENCE

Deliver the best outcomes and highest-quality service through the dedicated effort of every team member.

_____

_____

_____

_____

_____

_____

_____

_____

_____

_____

_____

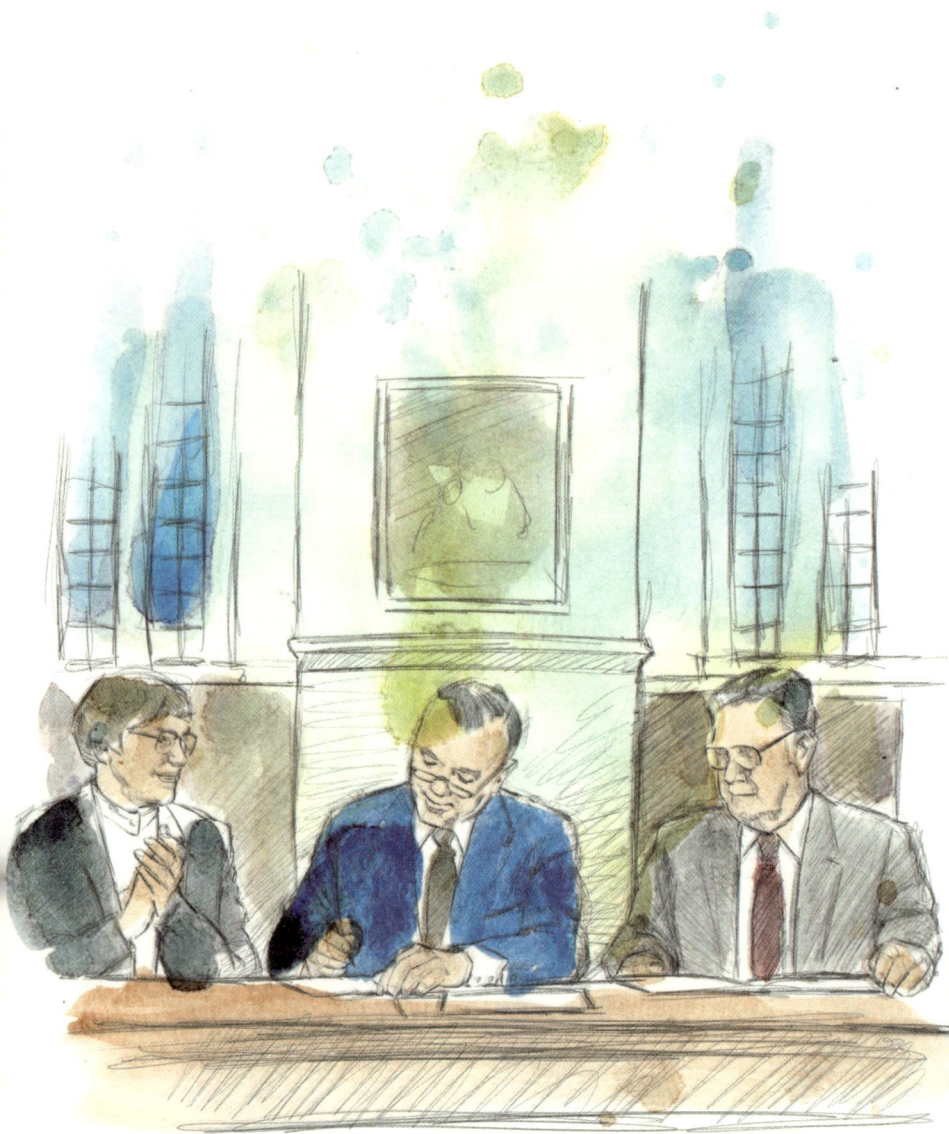

Saint Marys Hospital, Mayo Clinic and
Rochester Methodist Hospital
formed a unified governance structure.

CHAPTER EIGHT

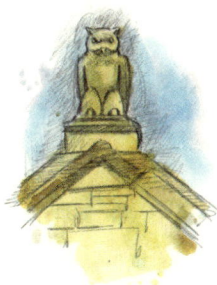

RESPECT

"A trusteeship for health."

— Governance Document

SUNLIGHT STREAMED INTO THE MITCHELL STUDENT CENTER OF MAYO Medical School on May 28, 1986. It brought a warm glow to a milestone event: Leaders representing Mayo Clinic, Saint Marys Hospital and Rochester Methodist Hospital signed a document that formalized their "historic existing relationships, creating a more fully integrated medical center under a single trusteeship." Building upon decades of collaboration, three separate organizations now came together as one.

Many factors drove the decision, which followed lengthy, wideranging discussions. Healthcare, always a personal relationship of patients with their physicians, nurses and other professionals, was increasingly drawn into economic and regulatory issues. Additional factors, including an aging population, advancing technology, competition from other healthcare providers and changes in American society, also played a role.

These forces would not abate. Indeed, they kept evolving and accelerating, a pattern that continues today. In response, Mayo's leaders turned to Mayo's values in order to set new directions that balanced the timeless commitment "to heal the sick and to advance the science" with the need for ongoing reinvention of how best to carry out that mission. Among the most important values was respect: placing the needs of the patient first and working to support the well-being of employees and colleagues.

First grants from the National Institutes of Health.

Mayo's value of respect stood in stark contrast to many practices in business and industry. In this era, takeovers, mergers, buyouts and acquisitions were common in the corporate world. The financial bottom line — for shareholders and for insiders who stood to reap huge profits — often was the determining force guiding decisions that affected multitudes of employees and consumers.

A respectful approach was vital when discussions

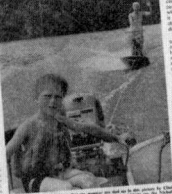

MAYOVOX

Dr. Osborn Dies at 38

Clinic Photographers to Host National Convention of BPA

'Better Prepared for Flu Than in 1918'–Magath

Grants Made

Mayo Association has been notified that two recent applications for research grants through the Department of Health, Education and Welfare have been approved.

Both grants are for research to be carried out in Dr. A. Albert's Endocrinology Laboratory. Titles of the projects are "Studies on the Pituitary Exophthalmogenic Hormone" and "Studies on Human Urinary Gonadotropin."

The Ruth and Frederic Mitchell Student Center welcomes medical students.

arose and decisions were made that were difficult and even painful. One early example was Mayo's decision in 1956 to begin accepting research funds from the National Institutes of Health. A decade later, the topic of whether Mayo Clinic should establish a medical school was hotly debated.

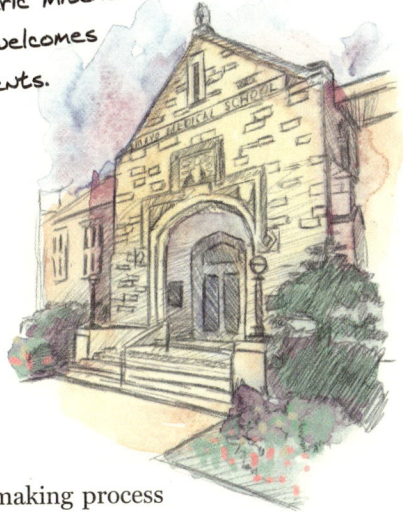

Mayo's consensus-based decision-making process ensured that individuals could have their say and diverse points of view could be explored. When the decisions were made, they were grounded in Mayo's traditional values. In announcing the acceptance of federal grants, Samuel Haines, M.D., chair of the Board of Governors, described "a moral responsibility ... with giving the best in medical care, and with doing our best in medical education and research." At the first convocation of Mayo Medical School in 1972, Dean Raymond Pruitt, M.D., said: "... the primary mission of our Mayo institutions, of our profession, of our science, of our new school is a mission on behalf of the humane."

When other large organizations evolved in this era, it often was because they went on a "shopping spree," acquiring businesses and entering industries far removed

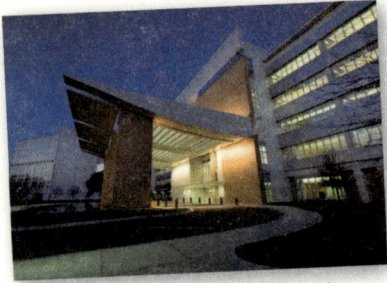

The Jacksonville, Florida, campus opened in 1986. The hospital (pictured) opened in 2008.

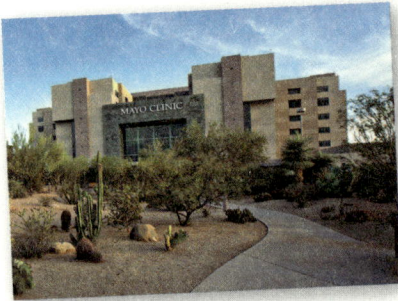

The Scottsdale, Arizona, campus opened in 1987. Mayo Clinic Hospital and the Phoenix campus (pictured) opened in 1998.

from their original mission. Culture clashes and economic dislocations often resulted. Mayo's leaders, by contrast, remembered Dr. Will's words: "We never have been allowed to lose sight that the main purpose to be served by the Clinic is the care of the sick."

This focus on serving patients kept Mayo Clinic grounded, but it also encouraged an entrepreneurial spirit that opened avenues Dr. Will never imagined. The early 1980s saw the start of "diversification," which included fundraising, the commercial application of Mayo's discoveries and intellectual property, the expansion of Mayo's reference laboratory system, and the publication of health information for consumers. After decades of avoiding the news media, Mayo began to share its message, as patients described their experience in receiving high-quality, compassionate care.

Across the generations, "Mayo Clinic" meant "an outpatient practice in Rochester, Minnesota." That definition changed as Mayo integrated with Saint Marys Hospital and Rochester Methodist Hospital in 1986 ... opened in Florida that year and in Arizona in 1987 ... developed Mayo Clinic Health System starting in 1992 and then Mayo Clinic Care Network in 2012. Respectful engagement was at the forefront. Quality of care, economic benefit, and expansion of scholarly activities in medical research and education are consistent measures of the respectful way that Mayo Clinic works with each of its communities.

MAYO CLINIC
HEALTH SYSTEM

Mayo Clinic Health System, which serves the Upper Midwest, was founded in 1992.

Respect continues to underscore the relationship between Mayo Clinic and the Franciscan Sisters. After the Second Vatican Council (1962-1965), fewer women entered religious life and some Sisters left Saint Marys Hospital. As administrators, Sister Mary Brigh Cassidy and Sister Generose Gervais graciously welcomed laypeople into positions of responsibility at the hospital.

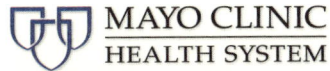

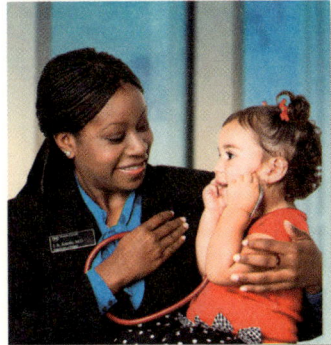

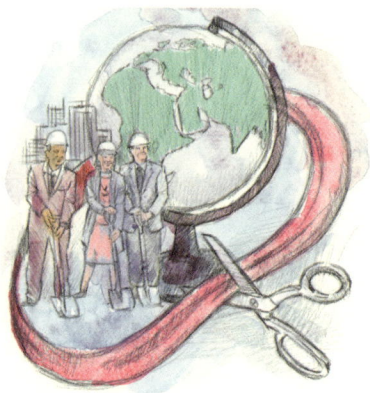

This, in turn, helped pave the way for a closer relationship with Mayo Clinic and an extension of the Franciscan spirit to Mayo colleagues beyond Saint Marys Hospital.

Throughout the process that began with the "trusteeship for health" document in 1986, the Franciscan Sisters and the people of Mayo Clinic have articulated and attempted to live out a series of values that set Mayo Clinic apart — while also providing an example that inspires organizations and people throughout the United States and around the world.

ENDNOTES

Page 57:   The statement about "historic existing relationships" is published in *25th Anniversary of Integration: Milestones of Trust*. **Rochester, Minnesota: Mayo Foundation for Medical Education and Research, 2011.**

Page 58:   "To heal the sick and to advance the science" is quoted in **Willius, p. 27.**

Page 59:   Samuel Haines, M.D., used the phrase "a moral responsibility" in a report entitled *Confidential Report to the Staff, November 24, 1956,* **p. 2. Mayo Clinic Archives.**

Page 59:   Raymond Pruitt, M.D., described the school's "primary mission" in *The Unending Adventure.* **Privately printed, no date, p. 25.**

Page 60:   "We have never been allowed to lose sight …" is included in **Willius, p. 45.**

CHECK YOUR COMPASS

RESPECT

Treat everyone in our diverse community, including patients, their families and colleagues, with dignity.

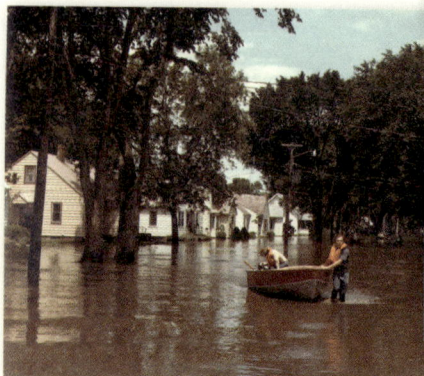

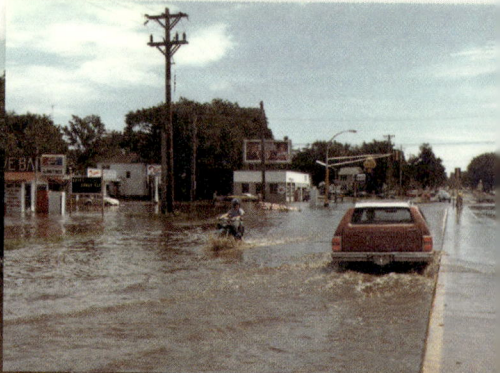

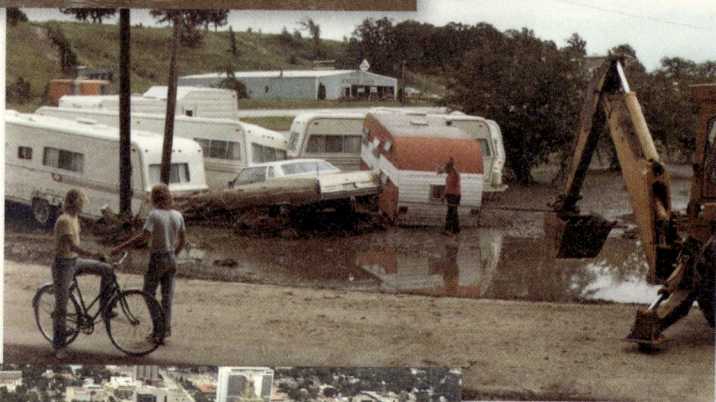

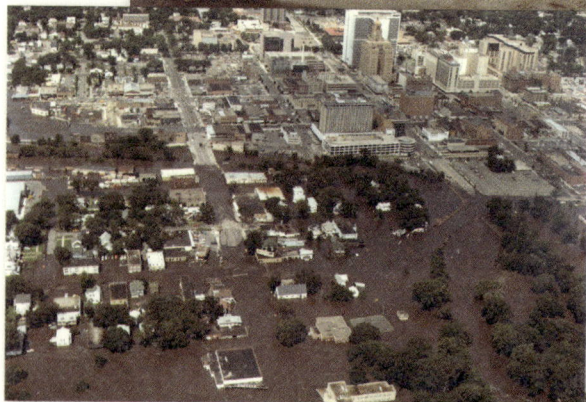

Flood! Rochester,
Minnesota,
July 5-6, 1978.

CHAPTER NINE

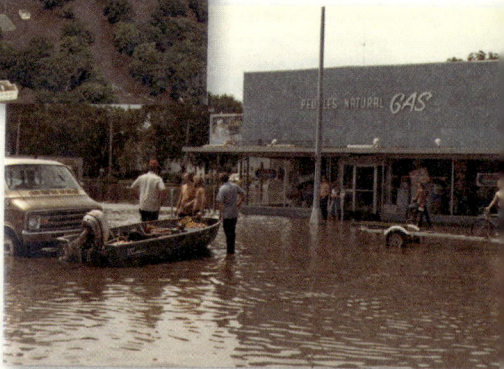

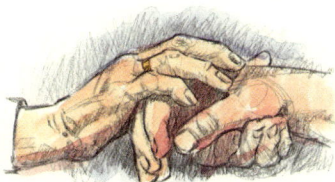

COMPASSION

"Values are caught, not taught."

— Sister Generose Gervais

T HE RAIN BEGAN AT 5:53 P.M. ON WEDNESDAY, JULY 5. NEARLY SEVEN inches fell in the next eight hours, inundating one-fourth of the city, causing $60 million in damage and claiming five lives. The flood of 1978 was the worst natural disaster to strike Rochester, Minnesota, since the tornado of 1883, which inspired the founding of Saint Marys Hospital.

By this time, Saint Marys was the largest private hospital in the United States. Filled with patients and staff, it also welcomed people who sought shelter from the storm and its aftermath. Fortunately, the hospital's chief administrator, Sister Generose Gervais, was equal to the crisis. She spent that night and the days that followed managing the hospital — not from her office, but by walking the halls and, as needed, by mopping the floor.

The comfort and compassion that Sister Generose demonstrated were indicative of her hands-on commitment and spirit of servant leadership, which have inspired generations of patients and colleagues alike. She received a papal commendation ... served as the first woman director of the Federal Reserve Bank in Minneapolis ... and was one of two women in her Master's in Health Administration Program at the University of Minnesota (earning straight A's), but she equally enjoyed talking about the crops, her beloved Minnesota Twins baseball team or activities on the sprawling Saint Marys campus.

Sister Generose grew up in southwestern Minnesota during the Dust Bowl years of the Great Depression on a farm with no electricity or running water. She entered the Franciscan congregation at age 18 and taught school during World War II. She earned a degree in home economics and entered Saint Marys Hospital as a dietetics intern. Soon she was tapped to serve as co-director of the Saint Marys School of Practical Nursing, followed by service as superior of the Saint Marys convent and assistant to Sister Mary Brigh Cassidy, the hospital's chief administrator.

In 1971, she became the fifth Franciscan Sister to lead the hospital. "Her insistence on economy and accountability kept Saint Marys financially strong during an era in which rising costs drained the coffers of

Sister Generose, left, reviewed construction plans with Sister Mary Brigh Cassidy.

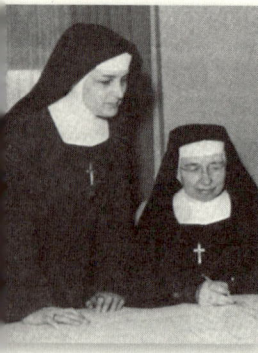

Bread & Butter Pickles

1 gal. cucumbers, fresh
washed, sliced thin, shaken down
4 cups onions, sliced & cut in pieces
1 green pepper, sliced into strips and
    cut in pieces
1 sweet red pepper, sliced into
    strips and cut in pieces
½ c. pickling salt

crushed ice
5 c. white sugar
5 c. cider vinegar
2 tbsp. mustard seed
2 tsp. celery seed
1½ tsp. tumeric
1½ tsp. ground cloves

. Mix cucumbers, onions, peppers and salt. Cover with crushed ice. Cover with towel; let stand 3 hours. Remove any ice and drain in colander. Put vinegar, sugar and spices in large kettle and place over high heat and stir. When sugar is dissolved, add cucumber mixture and stir. Bring quickly to full rolling boil, stirring carefully often enough to cook evenly. Dish immediately into hot sterilized jars and seal. (Do not overcook.) Makes 7 to 8 pints.

Sister Generose

many hospitals."

Indeed, these were years of expansion. The Mary Brigh Building, dedicated in 1980, was the largest hospital project in Minnesota's history to date. "She was as comfortable with the complexity of blueprints as she was with canning fruit," noted a colleague who worked closely with her. "She knew every corner of the hospital and how each space could best be used."

The bankers and lawyers who were evaluating the issuance of bonds for the construction project asked to review Saint Marys' contract with Mayo Clinic. "We don't have a contract," Sister Generose replied. "They couldn't believe it," she later recalled. They asked,

Sister Generose shared a favorite recipe.

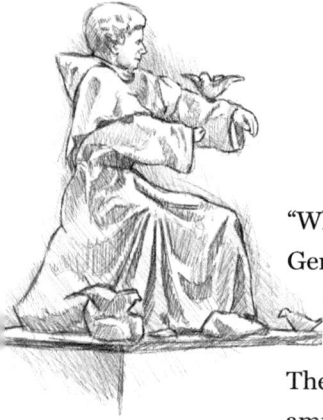

St. Francis
of Assisi —
statue at
Saint Marys.

"What do you do when you have a problem?" Sister Generose explained: "Those who are concerned with the problem get together, discuss possible solutions, choose what seems best and set about doing it." They commented: "This has to be the greatest living example of trust in the world, for two organizations of such size and complexity to work together like this." For Sister Generose, however, this relationship is a natural extension of the handshake and mutual trust between Dr. William Worrall Mayo and Mother Alfred Moes in the 19th century.

At Mayo Clinic, one of the most frequently quoted aphorisms of Sister Generose is "No money, no mission." But, she was quick to add, there is an equally important corollary: "No mission, no need for money." For Sister Generose, in fact, mission came first.

One of her most significant contributions to that mission is the Poverello Foundation, whose purpose is "to ease the burden for patients who need financial support for the care they received at Saint Marys Hospital." The foundation is named for St. Francis of Assisi, who was known as "Il Poverello" or "the little poor man." While the Poverello Foundation provides important financial support, Sister Generose believed that its enduring impact is

Sister Generose often met with Mayo Clinic employees.

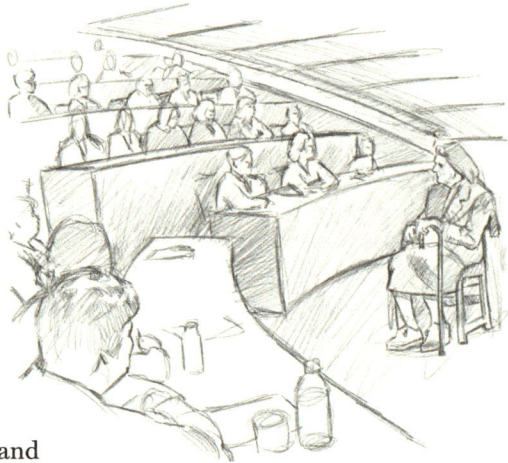

the sense of hope and renewal that recipients experience.

Sister Generose was the last Franciscan to serve as chief administrator of Saint Marys Hospital. In 1986, Saint Marys, Rochester Methodist Hospital and Mayo Clinic formalized their relationship by establishing a single governance structure, "a trusteeship for health." Continuing this momentum, in 2014 the two hospitals united into a single legal entity called Mayo Clinic Hospital — Rochester. To honor the hospital's heritage, its two geographic locations retain the historic names of Saint Marys Campus and Methodist Campus.

Dr. Charlie said his father "never really did retire," and, like

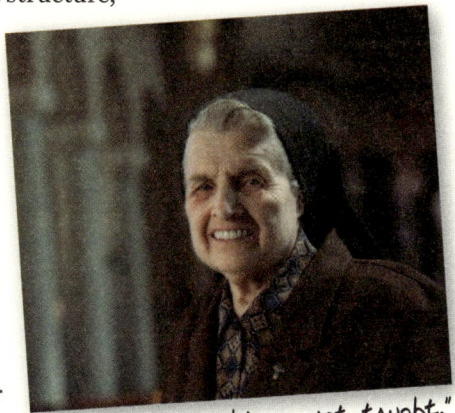

"Values are caught — not taught."

Dr. William Worrall Mayo, the same may be said of Sister Generose, who remained active at Saint Marys until her death in 2016. She was one of the most sought-after speakers at Mayo Clinic, often address-

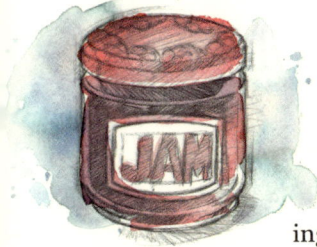

Selling preserves to raise funds for the Poverello Foundation.

ing employees who were born after she stepped down as chief administrator of Saint Marys in 1986.

Sister Generose was pleased to accept these invitations, but she deftly turned attention away from herself. "Values are caught, not taught" was one of her frequent maxims, and she reminded colleagues of what a beggar said to St. Francis many years ago: "Be sure thou art as good as the people believe thee to be, for they have great faith in thee."

Bringing that message home to her audience, she gently urged: "Be sure you are as good as the people think you are, for they have great faith in you — and you are *Mayo Clinic*."

ENDNOTES

Page 65:   Description of the flood comes from the National Weather Service Forecast Office, La Crosse, Wisconsin. Online report: *Summer of 1978: Flash Floods No. 2, July 5-8, 1978: Austin and Rochester, MN.*

Pages 66-70:   Summary of background, education and ministry of Sister Generose Gervais is included in **Whelan, Volume Two, p. 175-178.** The founding and mission of the Poverello Foundation is covered in **Whelan, Volume Two, pp. 218-219.**

Pages 69-70:   *A Conversation with Sister Generose: January 30 and February 11, 2014.* **Mayo Clinic Archives.** Videotaped interview.

Page 70:   Sister Generose paraphrased the beggar's admonition to St. Francis. *Ibid.*

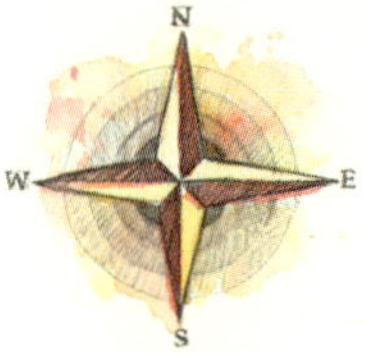

CHECK YOUR COMPASS

COMPASSION

Provide the best care, treating patients and family members with sensitivity and empathy.

_____

_____

_____

_____

_____

_____

_____

_____

_____

_____

_____

_____

_____

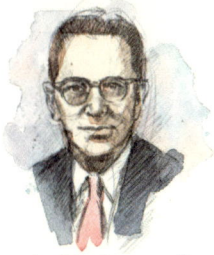

Harry A. Blackmun, J.D.

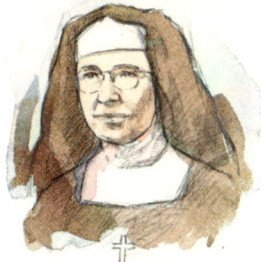

Sister Mary Brigh Cassidy

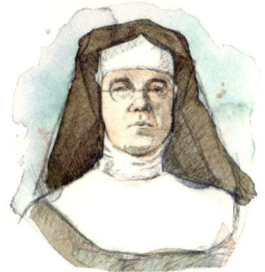

Sister Joseph Dempsey

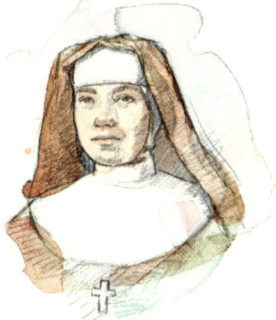

Sister Domitilla
DuRocher

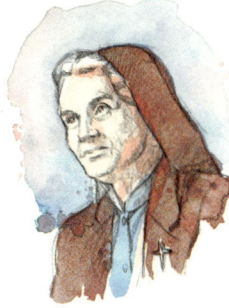

Sister Generose Gervais

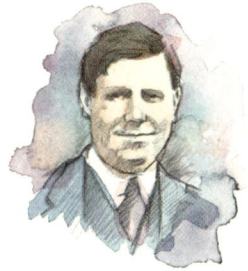

Harry J. Harwick

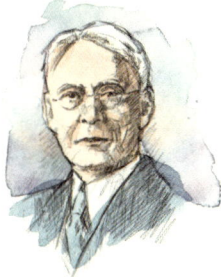

John H. Kahler

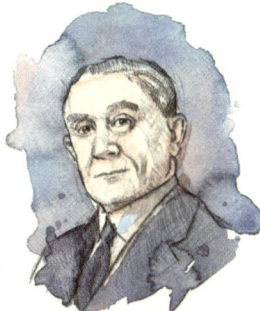

Charles H. Mayo, M.D.

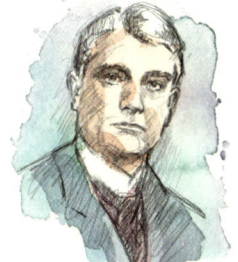

William J. Mayo, M.D.

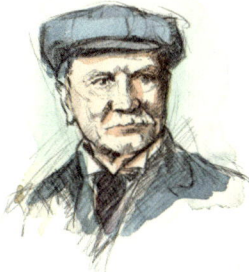

William Worrall Mayo, M.D.

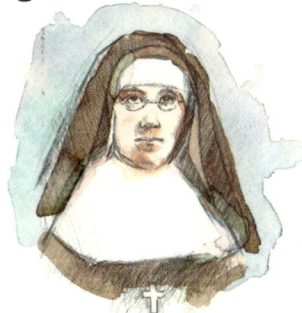

Mother Alfred Moes

CHAPTER 10

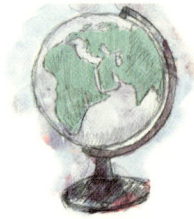

FRIENDS ALONG THE JOURNEY

"The glory of medicine is that it is constantly moving forward ..."

— Dr. Will Mayo

ONE OF THE IMPORTANT ASPECTS OF PILGRIMAGE IS THE COMMUNITY of people you meet along the way, as well as those who accompany you on your path. Among the many people who have lived the values and shaped the history of Mayo Clinic, this book includes the following individuals. May you sense their presence and extend their vision in your own journey.

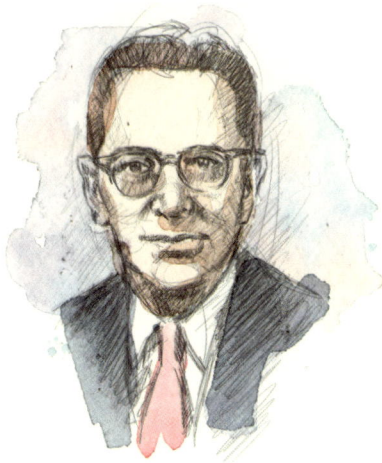

HARRY A. BLACKMUN, J.D.

ORN IN ILLINOIS, HARRY BLACKMUN GREW UP IN ST. PAUL, MINNE-
sota, where a grade school classmate was Warren Burger, future
member of the Mayo Clinic Board of Trustees and chief justice of the
United States Supreme Court. Harry Blackmun attended Harvard College on a scholarship, followed by Harvard Law School.

After establishing a successful legal practice in the Twin Cities, he
served as resident counsel of Mayo Clinic from 1950 to 1959, where he
played a leadership role in establishing Rochester Methodist Hospital.
Harry Blackmun often said "the happiest years" of his career were in
Rochester. He was appointed judge of the Eighth Circuit Court of Ap-
peals in 1959, followed by appointment to the United States Supreme
Court, where he served from 1970 to 1994.

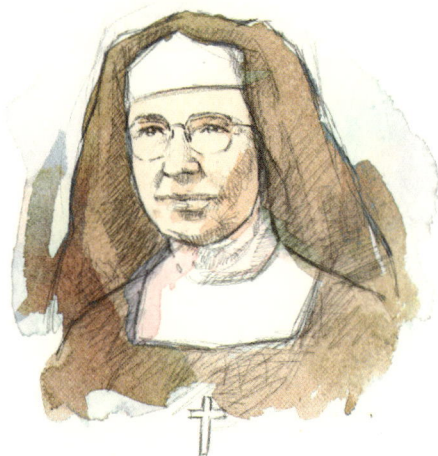

SISTER MARY BRIGH CASSIDY

A CONSUMMATE ADMINISTRATOR FOR 22 YEARS, SISTER MARY BRIGH was a warm, approachable woman who walked the halls of the hospital at the end of every day, visiting patients and encouraging staff. One colleague described her as being "a gentlewoman with quiet Irish chutzpah."

Sister Mary Brigh valued the broad perspective of lay colleagues. When the number of Sisters working at the hospital decreased and as Sisters retired from supervisory positions, she appointed laypeople in their places. Sister Mary Brigh created the hospital's first Board of Trustees, consisting of seven laypersons and eight Franciscans. Her bold initiatives ensured the hospital's growth and stability, and strengthened the Mayo-Franciscan partnership.

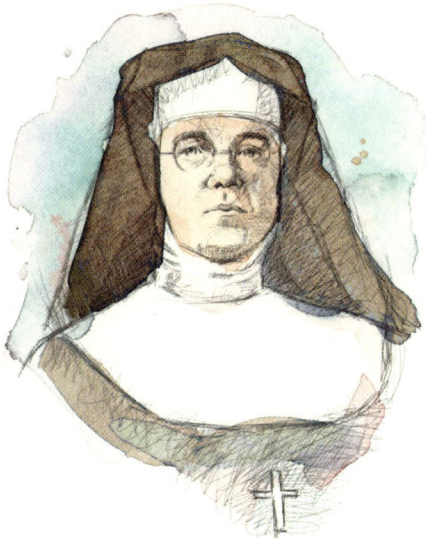

SISTER JOSEPH DEMPSEY

SISTER JOSEPH BEGAN 50 YEARS AS A NURSE AND HOSPITAL SUPERIN-tendent shortly after Saint Marys opened. Her unusual ability as a surgical nurse prompted Dr. Will to choose her over a physician as his first assistant. They often worked before a gallery of visiting surgeons. Dr. Will explained the procedure while Sister Joseph went on with the operation. Dr. Will said, "Of all the splendid surgical assistants I have had, she easily ranks first."

The hospital was the Sisters' home, and hospitality was the rule. Sisters treated each patient and employee with friendliness and respect. New employees received training from the Sister in charge of their area. They also learned about the hospital's mission, most often translated as "the patient comes first." A bond of shared dedication among the Franciscans and their lay colleagues made them in many respects like one family.

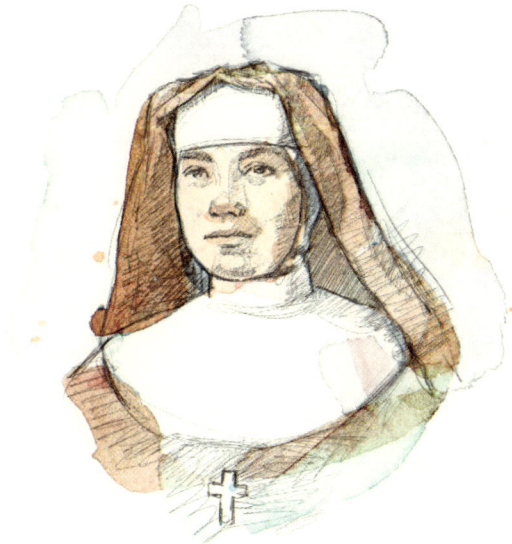

SISTER DOMITILLA DUROCHER

A NATIONAL LEADER IN NURSING, SISTER DOMITILLA BECAME ADMIN-istrator of Saint Marys Hospital in 1939. The first American Sister to receive a nursing degree, she graduated from Columbia University. Her background in the basic sciences and administration served the medical center well.

As the nation braced itself for World War II, Sister Domitilla acted with dispatch to improve patient services and reorganize for greater efficiency. Her initiatives brought sweeping changes, from new departments to a state-of-the-art medical wing. When Mayo physicians requested laboratories in the new building for clinical trials, Sister Domitilla directed architects to design patient floors and research laboratories in close proximity. The legacy of these laboratories lives on in Mayo's remarkable contributions to medical research, including the isolation of cortisone and its effective treatment of rheumatoid arthritis.

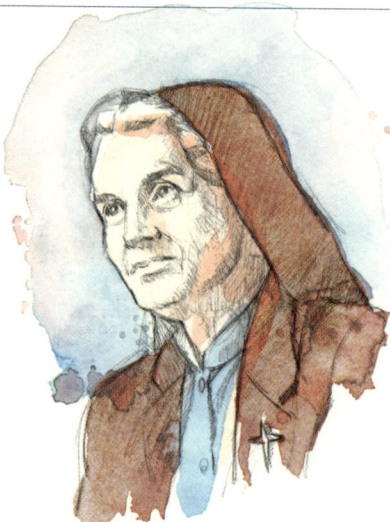

SISTER GENEROSE GERVAIS

SISTER GENEROSE COMBINED AN OPENNESS TO SERVE WITH THE ABILITY to master almost any assignment. From 1971 to 1986, she was the fifth Sister and last Franciscan chief administrator of Saint Marys Hospital.

One of her memorable contributions is the Poverello Foundation, which helps patients who need financial support for the care they received. Named for St. Francis of Assisi ("Il Poverello" or "the little poor man"), the foundation helps about 400 persons each year.

Until her death in 2016, Sister Generose was one of the most sought-after speakers at Mayo Clinic. With stirring examples, she told how ordinary and heroic acts of staff put the patient first and helped bring the medical center through dark times. "Their overriding goal was to give each patient the best care in the world," she said. "Each of you has that same goodness and strength. Use it to serve every patient and each other."

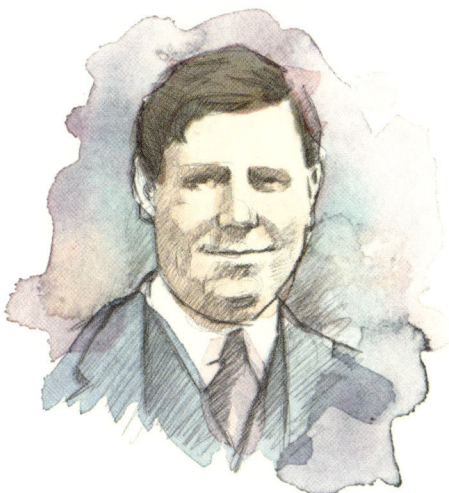

HARRY J. HARWICK

H ARRY HARWICK JOINED THE MAYO MEDICAL PRACTICE IN 1908, ON his 21st birthday. In the course of a 44-year career, he pioneered the profession of medical administration, uniting sound business principles with the medical ideals of the Mayo brothers. The collegial relationship that he shared with Dr. Will Mayo established the principle of physician-administrator collaboration, which is one of the enduring strengths of Mayo Clinic.

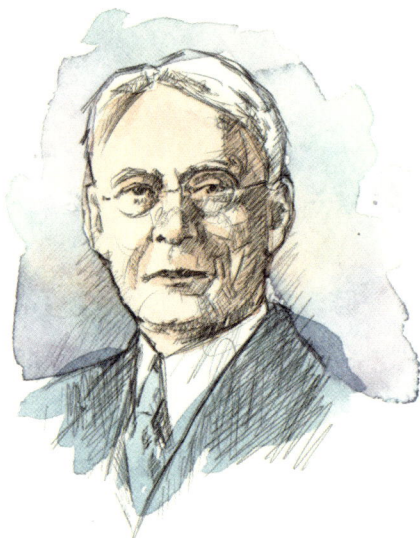

JOHN H. KAHLER

A N ENTREPRENEURIAL BUSINESS LEADER AND CLOSE FRIEND OF THE
Mayo brothers, John Kahler responded to acute demands for hospital beds and patient amenities to support the growing Mayo practice.

Based upon his observations in Europe, in 1907 he opened a combined hospital-hotel where patients could recuperate and family members could stay, all in close proximity to the Mayo medical offices. His enterprise grew into a network of hospitals and related services. After World War II, the Kahler Corporation decided to focus on the hospitality industry. Rochester Methodist Hospital was established to provide hospital care in downtown Rochester.

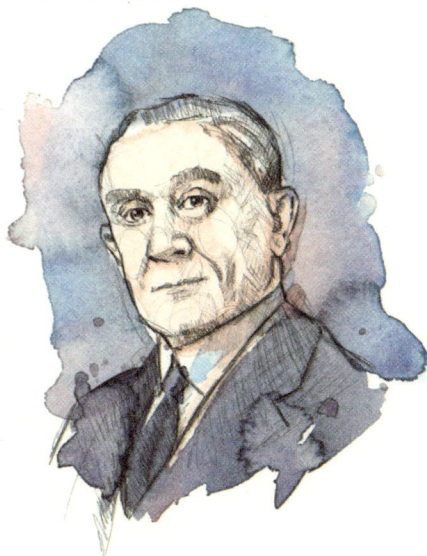

CHARLES H. MAYO, M.D.

THE YOUNGER MAYO BROTHER, KNOWN AS DR. CHARLIE, WAS BORN in Rochester, Minnesota, in 1865. Known for his warm, affable nature, he graduated from what is now the medical school of Northwestern University and specialized in head and neck surgery. Dr. Charlie married Edith Graham, R.N., the first professionally educated nurse in Rochester, who taught nursing skills to the Sisters of St. Francis. Dr. Charlie and Edith made Mayowood, their country estate, a center of hospitality.

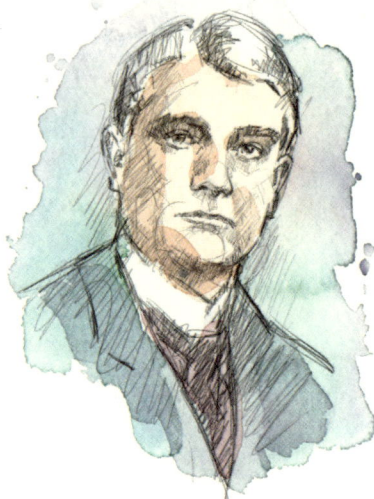

WILLIAM J. MAYO, M.D.

D R. WILL, THE ELDER MAYO BROTHER, WAS BORN IN LE SUEUR, Minnesota, in 1861, before his family moved to Rochester. A graduate of the University of Michigan, Dr. Will specialized in gastric surgery. Like his brother, he received honors from throughout the United States and around the world and served as president of the American Medical Association.

An excellent administrator as well as an acclaimed surgeon and educator, Dr. Will married Hattie Damon, his childhood friend. They often entertained guests on their riverboats as well as at their home. In 1938, they donated their residence to Mayo Foundation as a meeting place "for the good of mankind." Dr. Will and Dr. Charlie as well as Sister Joseph Dempsey, their close colleague and longtime superintendent of Saint Marys Hospital, all died within a few months of each other in 1939. Their shared legacy is the spirit of teamwork and service at Mayo Clinic.

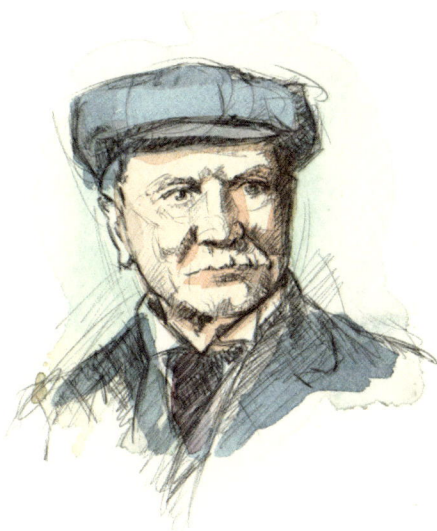

WILLIAM WORRALL MAYO, M.D.

BORN NEAR MANCHESTER, ENGLAND, IN 1819, W.W. MAYO IMMIGRATED to the United States as a young man, earned two medical degrees when most physicians had no formal education, and settled his young family in Rochester, Minnesota, during the Civil War. Active in civic affairs and possessed of a strong social conscience, he was one of the leading physicians in Rochester when a tornado devastated the frontier community in 1883.

The collaboration of Dr. Mayo with Mother Alfred Moes in the aftermath of that tragedy led to Mother Alfred's bold vision that the Sisters of St. Francis would fund construction of a hospital and serve as nurses if he and his sons would provide the medical care. The handshake that sealed their agreement symbolizes the Mayo Clinic Values.

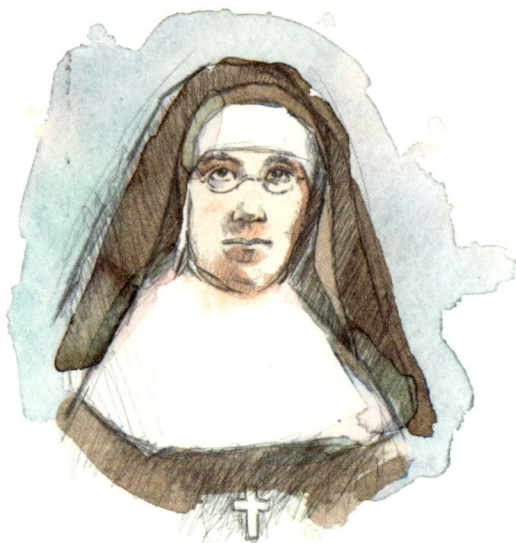

MOTHER ALFRED MOES

MOTHER ALFRED, BORN IN LUXEMBOURG, FOUNDED TWO TEACHING congregations and a score of schools across the Midwest. In 1883, a tornado in Rochester convinced her that the community needed a hospital. Dr. W.W. Mayo and his sons agreed to collaborate. As medical science moved forward with new momentum, the Franciscan Sisters and the Doctors Mayo shared the resolve to incorporate medical advances.

At Saint Marys Hospital, the Sisters created an inviting, homelike environment and served meals of highest quality. Sister Joseph Dempsey recalled that Mother Alfred "sometimes worked continuous shifts of one day and night and another day. She carried water from the basement to the upper floors, delivered trays of food to patients' rooms, shoveled coal and pinked oilcloth to make covers for the washstands in patients' rooms." Inspired by her extraordinary dedication, "Values are caught, not taught" became the maxim for patient care at Saint Marys Hospital.

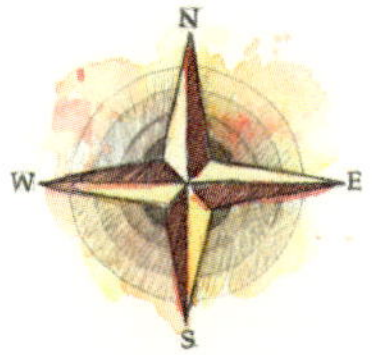

CHECK YOUR COMPASS

FRIENDS ALONG THE JOURNEY

Who are your "role models and soul models" at Mayo Clinic? How have they inspired you?

_____

_____

_____

_____

_____

_____

_____

_____

_____

_____

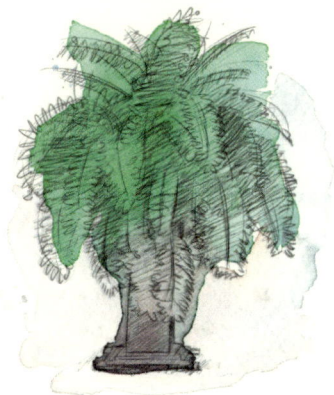

At Mayo Clinic, plants and
flowers are part of the
healing process.

ACKNOWLEDGMENTS

I T IS A PLEASURE TO THANK THE PEOPLE WHO SUPPORTED THE CREATION of this book.

Benefactors Gerald and Henrietta Rauenhorst provided generous funding that made the publication possible. Sister Marlene Pinzka, Ph.D., and Sister Jean Keniry served with us on the committee that has administered the Rauenhorst gift to the Rochester Franciscans since 2007. Leaders of the Mayo Clinic Values Council — Robert Brown, Jr., M.D., Sister Tierney Trueman, Linda Matti and Ann Pestorious — advocated for the book and its associated online content. The illustrations of James Rownd contributed significantly to the volume's appearance and character. Kristi Hunter helped identify and locate historical images. Art directors Karen Barrie and Connie Brooks brought the project to life through design and production management. Lea Dacy, Jeanne Klein and Francine Hedberg provided editorial judgment and proofreading skills in their reading of the text. Matthew Russell and Sue Grooters facilitated review by John Noseworthy, M.D. Jennifer Conrad provided administrative support. We are grateful for the collaboration of the W. Bruce Fye Center for the History of Medicine (Mayo Clinic Archives) under the leadership of Christopher Boes, M.D., and Renee Ziemer; Sister Lauren Weinandt, archivist of Saint Marys Hospital; and Sister Mary Lonan Reilly, Ph.D., archivist emerita of the Rochester Franciscans. Judith Osborne and Ronald Ward devoted expertise to the production process. Kenna Atherton and Christopher Frye secured ISBN and Library of Congress numbers. To these individuals and all "friends of the project," whose encouragement has sustained us, we express gratitude for helping us share the story of Franciscan-Mayo collaboration across the generations.

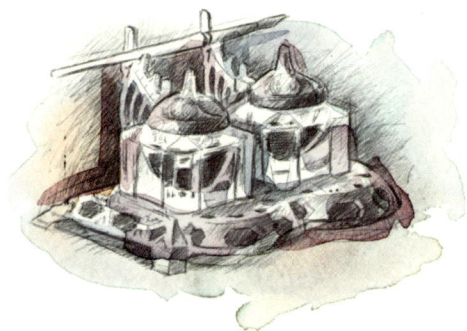

ABOUT THE AUTHORS

SISTER ELLEN WHELAN, PH.D.

SISTER ELLEN WHELAN, PH.D., FOLLOWED IN THE FOOTSTEPS OF FOUR of her aunts when she joined the Sisters of St. Francis of Rochester, Minnesota. An educator, she received a doctorate in history from Syracuse University. Sister Ellen was associated with Saint Marys Hospital and Mayo Clinic in a wide range of roles, among them serving as chair of the Saint Marys Hospital Sponsorship Board, predecessor of the Mayo Clinic Values Council. Sister Ellen was the author of the *The Sisters' Story: Saint Marys Hospital – Mayo Clinic.* Volume One covers the period from 1889 to 1939; Volume Two covers 1939 to 1980.

MATTHEW D. DACY

MATTHEW D. DACY RECEIVED THE B.A. IN HISTORY FROM RIPON College and the M.A. in journalism from the University of Missouri. He was a Rotary Foundation scholar in Jerusalem, Israel, prior to joining Mayo Clinic in 1984. Matt serves as director of the Heritage Hall museum, chair of the Heritage Days program and executive producer of the Heritage Film series. He is the author and editor of books about the history and culture of Mayo Clinic as well as the website *history.mayoclinic.org.*

ABOUT THE ILLUSTRATOR

JAMES E. ROWND

JAMES E. ROWND EARNED A DEGREE IN COMMERCIAL ART FROM HENNEPIN Technical College. He worked for more than 20 years in the fields of advertising and editorial art in the Twin Cities. Since joining Mayo Clinic in 2001, he has specialized in editorial art in the medical setting, using his skills to bring institutional concepts and strategic initiatives to life through visual expression. Among his signature projects were Mayo Clinic's vision for leadership in the year 2020 and the exterior of a mobile exhibit that traveled to cities throughout the United States as part of the Mayo Clinic Sesquicentennial.

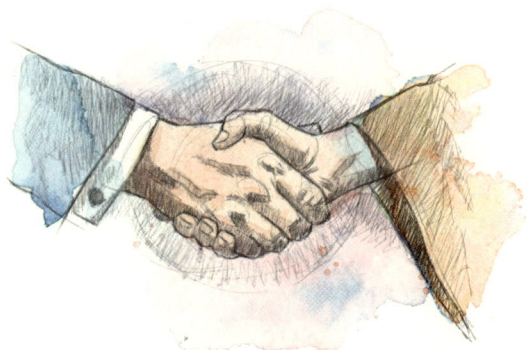

FOR MORE INFORMATION
history.mayoclinic.org